# BENIGN BREAST DISEASE

EDITED BY

James A. Smallwood MS, FRCS

and

Irving Taylor MD, ChM, FRCS
Department of Surgery
Southampton General Hospital
Southampton

with 12 contributors

Urban & Schwarzenberg • Baltimore

Edward Arnold
A division of Hodder & Stoughton
Mill Road, Dunton Green,
Sevenoaks, Kent TN13 2YA

Distributed in North America by
Urban & Schwarzenberg, Inc.
7 E. Redwood Street
Baltimore, Maryland 21202
USA

**NOTICES**

The Editors, Authors, and the Publisher of this work have made
every effort to ensure that the drug dosage schedules herein are
accurate and in accord with the standards accepted at the time of
publication. The reader is strongly advised, however, to check the
product information sheet included in the package of each drug he
or she plans to administer to be certain that changes have not been
made in the recommended dose or in the contraindications for
administration.

The publishers have made an extensive effort to trace original
copyright holders for permission to use borrowed material. If any
have been overlooked, it will be corrected at the first reprint.

**Library of Congress Cataloguing-in-Publication Data**

Benign breast disease/edited by J. A. Smallwood and I. Taylor with
    12 contributors.
        p.      cm.
    Includes bibliographical references.
    ISBN 0-8067-1891-9: $50.00 (est.)
    1. Breast—Diseases.      I. Smallwood, J. A. (James A.), 1952–
II. Taylor, Irvin.
    [DNLM: 1. Breast Diseases.   WP 840 B4673]
RG491.B46      1989
618.1'9—dc 20
DNLM/DLC
for Library of Congress

ISBN 0-8067-1891-9

Typeset in 10/11 pt Paladium by Colset Private Limited, Singapore
Printed and bound in Great Britain

# Contents

# List of Contributors

**R.W. Blamey** *MD, FRCS* Professor of Surgical Science, City Hospital, Nottingham.

**U. Chetty** *MS, FRCS* Senior Lecturer, University Department of Surgery, The Royal Infirmary Edinburgh.

**J.M. Dixon** *MD, FRCS* (Ed) Senior Lecturer in Surgery, University Department of Surgery, Edinburgh.

**I.S. Fentiman** *MD, FRCS* Consultant Surgeon, Clinical Oncology Unit, Guy's Hospital, London.

**W.D. George** *MS, FRCS* Professor of Surgery, Western Infirmary, Glasgow.

**P.B. Guyer** *MD, MS, FRCR, FRCP* Consultant Radiologist, Southampton General Hospital, Southampton.

**J. Hughes** *MRCP, MRCPsych.* Senior Research Fellow in Psychiatry, University of Southampton.

**J.A.E Hobby** *BSc, FRCS* Consultant Plastic Surgeon, Odstock Hospital, Salisbury.

**D.L. Page** *MD* Professor of Pathology, Vanderbilt University, Tennessee.

**P.E. Preece** *MD, FRCS* Senior Lecturer in Surgery, Ninewells Hospital, Dundee.

**K. Rogers** *MSc, FRCS* Senior Lecturer in Surgery, Northern General Hospital, Sheffield.

**J. A. Smallwood** *MS, FRCS* Lecturer in Surgery, University Surgical Unit, Southampton.

**I. Taylor** *MD, ChM, FRCS* Professor of Surgery, University Surgical Unit, Southampton.

# Benign breast disease – an introduction to the problem

Benign breast disease is an 'umbrella' term given to a wide spectrum of common non-malignant disorders of the female breast. Although the term 'benign' is correct in strictly pathological terms it nevertheless fails to convey the significant levels of discomfort, stress, and anxiety often produced.

Most women suffer from breast symptoms at some time during their life; in only a relatively small proportion, however, are the symptoms – or at least the patients' perception of the symptoms – sufficient to warrant medical consultation. Following referral, over 90% of such cases will ultimately have a benign condition.

The main concern of the patient – and indeed the clinician – rests with exclusion of malignancy. Having achieved this, management moves towards both specific therapy if required and 'active' reassurance.

There are several benign breast conditions usually associated with discreet abnormalities – for example, breast abscess, duct papilloma and plasma cell mastitis – which can without reservation be classified as 'disease'. Similarly, there are other often more 'generalised' conditions which are so common and of uncertain histological identity that they may more correctly be described as aberrations of normality, such as painful nodularity or mastalgia. In general, surgical excision of such lesions should be avoided unless real doubt exists as to the correct diagnosis; detailed reassurance and occasionally endocrinological manipulation are all that is required.

With the advent of national breast screening programmes the recognition of abnormalities on imaging will become even more important. Traditionally this has involved X-ray mammography but other techniques for assessment – for example, ultrasonography – will become more commonplace. It is incumbent upon radiologists and clinicians to recognise early invasive or *in situ* lesions with sufficient confidence to avoid excessive and unnecessary biopsies. It is also important that other benign lesions with an increased risk of future malignant change are recognised in biopsy material – for example, atypical lobular and ductal hyperplasia. Little is known at present of the natural history of breasts from which these lesions have been excised and less is known of how they should be treated or followed up; their study may also prove invaluable in the understanding of malignant transformation.

In 1985 and 1987 Southampton hosted two conferences on benign breast disease, and one of the major problems that emerged was the plethora of confusing nomenclature, much of which was meaningless. Most of the reviewers of the subjects discussed in this book, all experts in their own fields, were contributors at these conferences and are participants in a working party that is designed both to rationalise terminology and produce a working classification of benign conditions. In accord with these authors we have been able to standardise terminology and define terms where appropriate so they mean the same throughout the book.

In conclusion, benign breast disorders have failed to attract either the interest or concern that they undoubtedly deserve. As an attempt to redress this situation we have collated in this book detailed reviews of all aspects of benign disease ranging from aetiology and pathology to their treatment.

J Smallwood
I Taylor
Southampton

# 1

# The normal breast

JA SMALLWOOD

## Introduction

One of the factors that has ensured the survival and earthly domination of mammals for over 160 million years has been the ability to provide a ready made and superior food for their young. This 'milk' is secreted from mammary glands that develop from an epithelial ridge or milkline that runs ventrally from the axilla to the inguinal region; it disappears at an early embryological stage but leaves a number of epithelial cell rests which approximate to the likely number of offspring resulting from pregnancy. In primates a single pair remains, which contrasts with the eight pairs in rodents; the greatest number is seen in a species of South American marsupial that grows 25 pairs. Apart from man little is known of the range of breast diseases within the mammal world; the dog and mouse are certainly known to suffer a predisposition to breast cancer.

Breast disease has been known since the time of Hippocrates but the existence of 'benign' disease as a separate entity was not appreciated until the studies of Astley Cooper[1] and Benjamin Brodie[2] in the 1850s. Since this time a huge volume of scientific and clinical data has appeared, which has been associated with a plethora of terminology. One effect of this has been confusion as to what lies within the bounds of normality, particularly with regard to histopathology. The basic changes that occur in the structure and function of the breast through reproductive life are well established, but what can and should be accepted as a variant or aberration from the normal rather than 'pathology' is not. The following describes what is generally accepted as normal gross and microscopic structure followed by a discussion of what may be regarded as within normal limits.

## Gross anatomy

The human mammary gland lies totally within the superficial fascia of the anterior and lateral chest wall between the second and sixth intercostal space, and between the anterior axillary line and the edge of the sternum. The form of the breast depends more on the amount of fat than of glandular tissue that predominates in its upper half and extends into the lower axilla. This projection may at times form a distinct mass and be mistaken for more serious disease.

It is common for breasts to be unequal in size but rare for them to be absent or rudimentary. Accessory breasts or nipples are common, however, and may occur in 1–2% of white races and up to 6% in both sexes of oriental races.

Accessory structures occur as one or any combination of the three components of the breast – its glandular and ductal parenchyma, the areola, and the nipple. The most common accessory structure is a small areola and nipple, and the most common sites are just below a normal breast or the lower axilla. Where glandular tissue exists it is subject to diseases found in normally placed breasts and fibroadenomas, cysts, and carcinomas have all been described.

In some mammalian species breasts are found outside the milk line notably the lemur (inguinal region) and the whale (labia majora). Such atypical positions have been described in man with the above sites being the most common. Ton and Shanmugaratnam[3] have recently described 15 cases of human vulval breasts. Other sites described in man include the shoulder, scapula, thigh, midthorax, and midabdomen.

## Blood and lymphatic supply

The breast receives blood predominantly from perforating branches of the internal mammary artery. There are four main perforators passing through the corresponding intercostal space of which the first two are usually the largest. The lateral side of the breast receives blood from branches of the axillary artery to a variable degree. Named branches which contribute include the highest thoracic artery, the pectoral branch of the thoraco-acromial artery, and the lateral thoracic and subscapular arteries. Finally there are small perforating branches which pass into the breast from the intercostal arteries through the pectoral muscles. Venous drainage follows the same routes through similarly named veins.

The lymphatic drainage is mainly important in malignant disease but is occasionally of interest in breast infections or when lymph nodes within the breast mimic discrete breast lumps. Many studies before that of Turner-Warwick[4] produced conflicting data about the direction of lymphatic flow, but his work – supported by that of Hasell *et al*[5] – showed that lymph flow in the normal breast is from superficial to deep rather than centripetally. Thus the valveless subepithelial plexus drains lymph from the skin into a deeper, valved, subdermal plexus. As with the subareola plexus which drains the areola and nipple, lymph passes deep within the breast among the ducts and lobules and then drains to the major lymph node groups which are found in the axilla and the internal mammary chain. To a lesser extent it also drains by intercostal routes to the posterior paravertebral group. The broad nodal groups do not drain specific zones of the breast as shown by Turner–Warwick[4]; using autoradiographic techniques he demonstrated that all parts of the breast drain into all groups but most of the lymph clearance will tend towards the closer group of nodes.

The axillary nodes are often said by pathologists to form three main groups or levels.[6] Level one nodes are lateral and inferior to pectoralis minor and include the lateral, subscapular, and pectoral groups. Level two nodes lie posterior to pectoralis minor and are predominantly the central group. Level three nodes lie medial and superior to pectoralis minor and represent the apical or infraclavicular groups (Fig. 1.1).

## Microscopic structure

The breast is composed of about 20 lobes each made up of epithelial and stromal elements that are composite and no tissue planes exist. In each lobe there are between 10 and 100 lobules that drain through ductules into a subsegmental duct and finally into a segmental duct (Fig. 1.2). Near the nipple these ducts expand into lactiferous sinuses which narrow down into the collecting duct that finally opens out at the nipple. Close to the end of the collecting duct the epithelium is stratified squamous as is the nipple skin, but elsewhere along the duct system (as far as and including the acini in the lobule) the epithelium is composed of two layers: an inner columnar or 'tall' cell layer, and an outer and often incomplete layer of myoepithelial cells. Both cells may therefore border the basement membrane (Fig. 1.3).

The nipple and areola have certain distinctive histological features: the

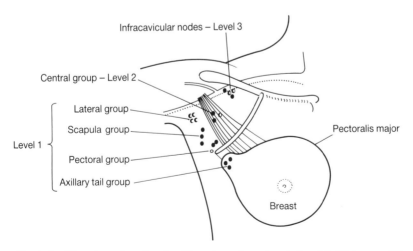

**Fig 1.1**   The three levels of axillary lymph nodes (after McDivitt *et al*[6]).

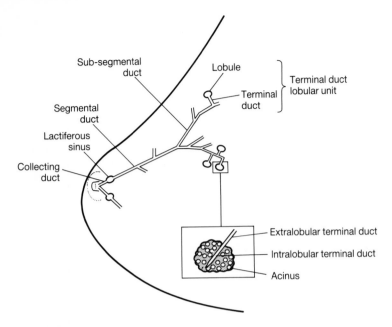

**Fig 1.2**   The ductal and lobular system of the breast.

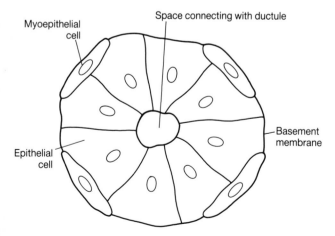

**Fig 1.3**   Epithelium of the duct and acinus.

epithelium is more deeply pigmented than normal skin and this is more marked in younger women whose oestrogen levels are elevated and in pregnant women. The nipple is hairless but there are often numerous follicles at the periphery of the areola. Within the skin there are well developed dermal papillae and numerous large sebaceous glands that tend to group around the openings of collecting ducts producing elevations. During pregnancy and subsequent lactation these glands enlarge further and are sometimes called Montgomery's tubercles. As well as sebaceous glands there are apocrine or sweat glands typical of those seen in the skin of the axilla and genital area. The subcutaneous tissue contains numerous irregularly arranged smooth muscle bundles in a bed of collagen stroma which, under sensory and endocrine stimulation, induce erection of the nipple.

A lobule with its draining ductule is commonly referred to as a terminal duct lobular unit. The lobule itself consists of between 10 and 100 acini bound together in fine vascular connective tissue (Fig. 1.4). The ductule tends to branch off the subsegmental ducts more or less at right angles and is usually short, being as long as the lobule diameter.[7] Some authors use the expression ductule or terminal ductule to describe the smallest lobular epithelial unit or acinus, and in these circumstances the terminal duct refers to what is described above as the ductule.[8]

In recent years attention has been focused on the stroma which has in some circumstances given clues to the origin of certain aberrations or disease states. The periductal stroma or connective tissue is distinct from that of the interlobular and intersegmental spaces by being loose, vascular, and more cellular; within the lobule this stroma is more abundant and even more cellular but unlike the periductal tissue it lacks elastic fibres. Elastic tissue surrounds the extralobular ductal system and increases in amount with age and parity. The 'lobular' origin of fibroadenomas is based partly on the

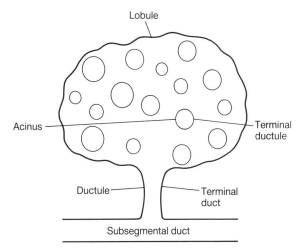

**Fig 1.4** Nomenclature of the lobule.

absence of any elastic tissue within these lesions.[7] The stroma and epithelium appear to be functionally interdependent, but the precise details have yet to be elucidated.

## Changes during the menstrual cycle

There is some dispute as to whether morphological changes can be appreciated during the different phases of the menstrual cycle but there is some evidence of subtle changes in some but not all the lobules at one time.[9, 10]

During the proliferative phase mitoses within the acini are initially quite common but they gradually lessen and the small luminal spaces slowly widen. In the secreting phase the lumina enlarge further and contain more secretions, while the lining epithelial cells develop microvilli and glycogen deposits. Late in this phase these cells exhibit true apocrine secretion with the 'pinching off' of portions of apical cytoplasm. During menstruation the lumina remain distended with granular secretions, but the cellular activity decreases.

It seems unlikely that there is any change in the number of lobules and acini in the premenstrual phase as suggested by the earlier work of Rosenberg.[11] Later studies by Haagensen[12] failed to show any such change, or even any recognisable alteration within the stroma. He suggested that any premenstrual change in breast density and size must be a consequence of blood or lymph engorgement or even increase in the extracellular fluid tension. More recent evidence from Preece *et al*,[13] who found little change in total body water content throughout the phases of the menstrual cycle, would not support this.

## Changes in the breast during pregnancy and lactation

Early in the first trimester of pregnancy lobular size increases only slightly, but the epithelial cells show marked changes with cytoplasmic vacuolation and prominent nucleoli. Mitoses are also seen. Towards the second trimester the lobules become markedly more swollen with larger and more numerous acini that are dilated with secretions. The epithelial cells show prominent organelle development and microvilli at the luminal surface.

In the last trimester these changes continue to increase, resulting in obliteration of the stroma. Myoepithelial cells do not proliferate as much but become elongated and stretched; the number of myofilament bundles increases, suggesting preparation for contractility. A yellowish fluid known as colostrum is frequently seen at the nipple during this phase.

With the onset of lactation the acini are even more distended with secretions, which fill out the ductal system. In the first 24 hours this secretion continues as colostrum but if breast feeding continues milk will appear on the second day. The longer the delay in breast feeding the longer the delay in the appearance of milk – often by 2 or 3 days.

# Breast involution

Involution begins as soon as lactation ceases, but also occurs at a much slower and more subtle rate in association with age. In the former case a complete return to the normal resting state by shrinkage and reduction of the lobules is rare, and some of the well developed lobules will persist.[14] Other changes that occur are seen in the description of age related involution below.

Morphometric studies[15] have suggested that lobular volume reduction with loss of epithelium begins at about the age of 30 and goes on until the early sixties. This is not solely dependent upon ovarian function as moderate or good lobular development can be found in over 75% of castrate women up to 15 years after the event.[14] The amount of resting epithelium over this period does not appear to be influenced by the number of pregnancies or by breast feeding. Whatever controls the complex mechanisms of involution, this can be shown to effect the lobules ducts and stroma at more or less the same time but such changes are not uniform and may vary from segment to segment.

## Lobular involution

The double layer epithelium of the acini and small ducts becomes flattened and the luminal space narrows to almost obliteration. The surrounding loose connective tissue slowly converts into dense hyaline collagen which tends to blend with the basement membrane and the surrounding background fibrous tissue. The lobular outline is thus lost and all that remains to suggest this original structure are epithelial remnants which may also finally disappear. The involuting process occasionally produces microcyst-like structures[16] which arise from acini that have coalesced. They too become replaced with dense fibrous tissue (Fig. 1.5).

## Ductal involution

Like the intralobular ducts, the interlobular ducts also disappear, but of the larger ducts that remain their walls become atrophic. There may be a patchy loss of elastic tissue but near the areola it is not uncommon to find an increase in surrounding elastic fibrous tissue. Little is known of the mechanisms of ductal involution but it may have some bearing on the aetiology of duct ectasia.

## Stromal involution

The supporting extralobular stroma of the breast also changes, in that it largely disappears to be replaced by adipose tissue. This replacement is variable and results in either a small atrophic or a large pendulous breast. It is the increase in fat content which accounts for the relative lucency on mammography of the post-menopausal breast. Although fat may imply an inert structure, significant aromatase activity has been found in fat from

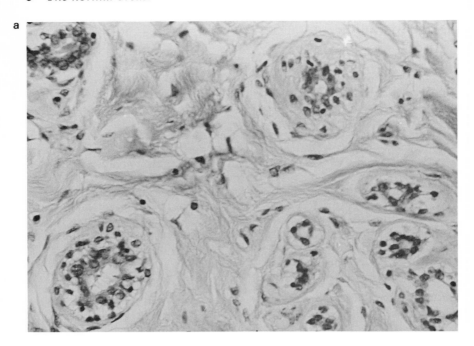

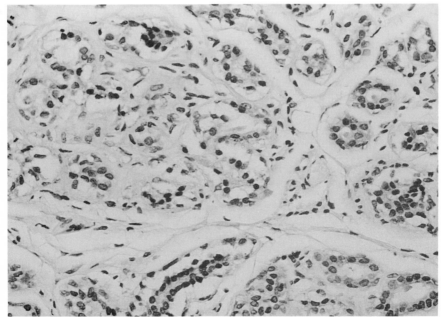

**Fig 1.5**  Breast microscopic appearances (a) during reproductive life and (b) after involution.

both normal and diseased breasts.[17] How this endogenous production of oestrogens influences structure and function is unknown.

Involution of the various elements within the breast occurs in a random fashion so that elements in one area of the breast may have disappeared while they remain prominent in another. This situation frequently leads to confusion both clinically and histopathogically where normal involution events may be constructed as abnormal or pathological.

## Normal or abnormal?

The dilemma about what should be considered as being within the range of normality has not been properly questioned in recent years. Although the breast appearances described above are 'normal' because they are consistently seen in most women, there are other appearances which are common, yet have frequently been ascribed 'disease states'. There are a number of reasons for this but one prime offender has been a long standing enthusiasm to relate histological patterns to breast cancer risk. Many such patterns have, through an erroneous association with cancer, been elevated to a pathological status that is undeserved. An obvious example here is that of 'fibroadenosis' which has an uncertain (if any) legitimate histological identity; it has nevertheless been repeatedly correlated with breast cancer, which of course has a well defined histological character. Furthermore, where careful studies have chosen specific histological patterns related to the fibroadenosis/cystic disease range no risk correlation with breast cancer has been found (see chapter 8).

An offender of equal significance has been the plethora of histological nomenclature which is so frequently used loosely by both pathologist and surgeon; it is possible to find over 30 synonyms or expressions for the condition known as 'fibroadenosis', most of which have been appropriated by clinicians to describe syndromes of symptons and signs. Much of the terminology was intended by histopathologists to be descriptive but has assumed a label implying disease; worse perhaps has been the knock-on effect of employing terms that have serious implications in disease of other organs – for example, dysplasia. In colonic and cervical disease, dysplasia has clear neoplastic connotations, whereas in the breast this essentially histological term has no histological identity. In the words of Azzopardi, 'Mammary dysplasia is perhaps one of the most objectionable and ill-defined terms in common use'.[19]

A less obvious factor that has hampered our perception of normality has been the attempts of pathologists to label biopsy material in a way that tries to justify the clinician's decision to biopsy. The correlation of static biopsy material with clinical symptoms and signs has rarely been validated by comparison with material from asymptomatic areas from the same or other breast; it also usually ignores the dynamic nature of breast glandular tissue as it undergoes the changes of development, involution, and the menstrual cycle. This was recognised as long ago as 1945 by Foote and Stewart[20] with regard to fibrocystic disease. They remarked that 'chronic cystic disease' of the breast is so engraved in the minds of some pathologists that the diagnosis of a locally excised portion of the breast amounts to a surgical-pathological reflex. More recent studies by both Parks[21] and Haagenson[22] have shown that supposed features of fibrocystic disease – microcysts, apocrine metaplasia, and adenosis – are so commonly seen that they should be regarded as normal; what is more, there is such a poor correlation with these changes and the signs and symptoms they are said to produce that Love[18] in 1982 coined the phrase 'fibrocystic disease of the breast is a non-disease'.

There is compelling evidence from many detailed studies that a number of changes in the breast are not pathological but within the normal range (Fig. 1.6). There is also another group of benign conditions that confer no cancer risk and are individually so common that to call them pathology or disease is at least debatable. Since they can be related to phases of reproductive life Hughes *et al*[23, 24] have recently proposed the acronym ANDI or 'abberations of normal development and involution'. This is particularly attractive as it allows for dynamic change such as that seen with cyclical mastalgia or nodularity and it promotes an idea of histogenesis or aetiology by implicating a reproductive phase. As many of these conditions (Fig. 1.6) impinge on the realm of normality a brief explanation of their position in the scheme will be presented.

### Fibroadenoma

The lack of elastic tissue within fibroadenomas is a signature of their lobular origin. In 1959 Parks[21] showed that hyperplastic lobules abound in the female breast and that these are indistinguishable histologically from the clinically detectable fibroadenoma. Why such hyperplasia should proceed

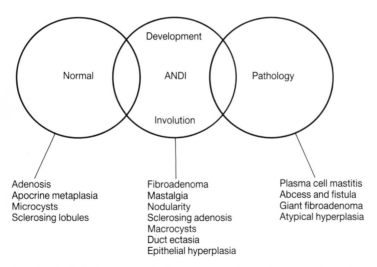

**Fig 1.6** Relationship of the normal breast with aberrations of normal development and involution and disease.

to clinically detectable fibroadenomas is unknown, but they tend to occur at a time of maximal hormonal stimulation and will even lactate should pregnancy supervene. In contrast to true neoplasms they rarely grow to more than 2-3 cm, may spontaneously regress[25] (about 25%), and more will involute at the time of the menopause. There is ample evidence therefore that small fibroadenomas are abberations of development rather than true pathology which should be reserved for the rarer giant fibroadenomas that exceed 4-5 cm.

## Mastalgia and nodularity

There is little dispute that premenstrual swelling and tenderness of the breast is a normal phenomenon without a discernable histological counterpart. The more severe cases that manifest themselves with significant mastalgia or nodularity, the type that is referred for specialist opinion, can be related to a subtle fault of pituitary/prolactin secretion, but once again there is no histological lesion. The use of the terms fibroadenosis, fibrocystic disease, and dysplasia are used by the clinician for convenience and by habit rather than science. The evidence of an endocrine aberration coupled with the severity of symptoms ideally places this condition within aberrations of normal development and involution.

## Sclerosing adenosis

While adenosis is so common that it is regarded as being within the sphere of normality there is some doubt as to whether the common type of sclerosing adenosis should be regarded as disease. The appearances fit with an aberration of involution where the process of stromal and lobular involution are occurring at times when there are still menstrual cycles with proliferative phases; it is not surprising that lobular elements should appear distorted by fibrous tissue. These findings are commonly seen in biopsy material but their incidence in asymptomatic normal breasts is unknown. Most types of sclerosing adenosis would qualify as an aberration of involution with the exception perhaps of sclerosing adenosis with pseudoinfiltration (infiltrating epitheliosis), where the relationship with malignant potential is uncertain.

## Duct ectasia

Whatever the cause of duct ectasia, the simple presence of dilated ducts often associated with nipple discharge is so common in perimenopausal or postmenopausal women that it should not be regarded as disease. As minor degrees of plasma cell periductal inflammation are frequently seen histologically it seems reasonable to classify this condition as an aberration of normal involution rather than as normal or pathological. Where symptomatic plasma cell mastitis, with or without suppuration, supervenes this is clearly in the realm of pathology.

## Epithelial hyperplasia

Simple lobular and ductal hyperplasia is very common in the pre-menopausal phase and has been reported in up to 60% of women over the age of 70.[26] Sloss[27] found this feature so common in autopsy breast specimens that he concluded 'its presence in the breast of women is insufficient to warrant such tissue being called disease'. The anxiety that simple hyperplasia may proceed to atypical hyperplasia with its recognised cancer risk[28] is legitimate but totally unproven. It seems reasonable to regard simple hyperplasia as an aberration of the normal involutionary process.

Since the suggestion of Hughes *et al*[23] of grouping conditions of uncertain pathological identity within 'aberrations of normal development and involution', a National Working Party has produced a new classification of benign conditions which embraces this concept. It is presented in Fig. 1.7, although the final classification has yet to be agreed; it will certainly be a valuable contribution both to our understanding and to the student for whom there is little in the standard surgical textbook.

## Conclusions

The structure of the normal breast changes throughout life and although basic anatomy and histology can be easily appreciated it seems that other features should be accepted within the normal range. Where the line should be drawn and the term 'disease' or pathology used is one which will attract continued debate; the distillation of a sensible classification and restricted nomenclature from the huge array of terminology and confusion will undoubtedly help.

## References

1. Cooper AP. *Anatomy and Diseases of the Breast*. Philadelphia, Lea and Blanchard, 1845.
2. Brodie BC. *Lectures Illustrative of Various Subjects in Pathology and Surgery*. London, Longman, 1846.
3. Ton SH, Shanmugaratnam K. Supernumerary mammary gland in the vulva. *Br Med J* 1962; ii: 1234.
4. Turner-Warwick RT. The lymphatics of the breast. *Br J Surg* 1959; 46: 574–82.
5. Hasell J, Smith J, Bentlage C, *et al*. Lymphatic drainage of the breast by vital dye staining and radiography. *Ann Surg* 1965; 162: 221–26.
6. McDivitt RW, Sherrat F, Beng JW. Tumours of the breast. In: *Atlas of Tumour Pathology II*. Washington, Armed Forces Institute of Pathology, 1968: 12.
7. Azzopardi J. Problems in breast pathology. In: (ed JL Bennington) *Major Problems in Pathology*. Vol. II. London, WB Saunders, 1987, pp. 14–15.
8. Sloane JP, Trott PA. In: *Biopsy Pathology of the Breast*. London, Chapman Hall, 1985, p. 4.
9. Farger H, Ree HJ. Cyclic changes of human mammary gland epithelium in relation to the menstrual cycle – an ultrasound study. *Cancer* 1974; 34: 574–85.
10. Vogel PM, Georgiade N, Fetter B *et al*. The correlation of histological changes in the human breast with the menstrual cycle. *Am J Pathol* 1981; 104: 23–24.
11. Rosenberg A. Über Menstrielle, dirsch das Corpus luteum bedingte Mammaverandeningen. *Frankfurt Zeitschrift fur Pathologie* 1922; 27: 466.

Common benign breast conditions falling into the classification of 'aberrations of normal development and involution' Aberrations of normal development and involution

| Stage (peak age in years) | Normal process | Aberration | Clinical presentation | Histology | Radiology | Disease |
|---|---|---|---|---|---|---|
| Early reproductive period (15–25) | Lobule formation | Fibroadenoma | Discrete lump | Fibroadenoma | Rounded density | Giant fibroadenoma Multiple fibroadenomas |
| | Stoma formation | Juvenile hypertrophy | Excessive breast development | | | |
| Mature reproductive period (25–40) | Cyclical hormonal effects on glandular tissue and stroma | Exaggerated cyclical effects | Cyclical mastalgia and nodularity generalised or discrete | No specific features | Non-specific density, generalised or local | |
| Involution (35–50) | Lobular involution (including microcysts, apocrine change, fibrosis, adenosis) | Macrocysts Sclerosing lesions | Discrete lumps Radiographic abnormalities | Benign cysts Sclerosing adenosis, radial scar | Rounded densities Microcalcification or distortion, or both | |
| | Ductal involution | Duct dilatation | Nipple discharge | Duct ectasia, periductal inflammation | Non-specific ductal thickening | Periductal mastitis with bacterial infection and abscess formation |
| | | Periductal fibrosis | Nipple retraction | Periductal inflammation and fibrosis | Non-specific ductal thickening | |
| | Epithelial turnover | Mild epithelial hyperplasia | Histological report | Mild epithelial hyperplasia | | |

Fig 1.7  New classification of benign breast conditions.

12. Haagensen CD. The normal physiology of the breasts. In: *Disease of the Breast*. 3rd ed. Philadelphia, WB Saunders, 1986, pp. 50–51.
13. Preece PE, Richards AR, Owen GM, Hughes LE. Mastalgia and total body water. *Br Med J* 1975; **iv**: 498–500.
14. Bonser GM, Dossett JA, Jul JW. In: *Human and Experimental Breast Cancer*. London, Pitman Medical, 1961.
15. Hutson SW, Cowen PN, Bird CC. Morphometric studies of age related changes in normal human breast and their significance for evolution of mammary cancer. *J Clin Pathol* 1985: **38**: 281–87.
16. Hayward JL, Parks AG. Alterations in the neuroanatomy of the breast as a result of changes in the hormonal environment. In: Currie AR. (ed) *Endocrine Aspects of Breast Cancer*. E & S Livingstone, 1958, London and Edinburg: 133–134.
17. O'Neill JS, Elton RA, Millar RW. Aromatase activity in adipose tissue from breast quadrants: a link with tumour site. *Br Med J* 1988; **296**: 741–43.
18. Love SM, Gelman RS, Silen W. Fibrocystic disease of the breast: a non-disease. *N Engl J Med* 1982; **307**: 1010–14.
19. Azzopardi J. Problems in breast pathology. In: *Major Problems in Pathology*. Vol. II. Philadelphia, WB Saunders, 1987, pp. 23–24.
20. Foote FW, Stewart FW. Comparative studies of cancerous versus non-cancerous breasts. *Ann Surg* 1945; **121**: 6–53.
21. Parks AG. The microanatomy of the breast. *Ann R Coll Surg Engl* 1959; **25**: 235–51.
22. Haagenson CD. The relationship of gross cystic disease of the breast and carcinoma. *Ann Surg* 1977; **185**: 375–76.
23. Hughes LE, Mansel RE, Webster DJT. Aberrations of normal development and involution (ANDI) – a new perspective in pathogenesis and nomenclature of benign breast disease. *Lancet* 1987; **ii**: 1316–18.
24. Hughes LE, Mansel RE, Webster DJT. ANDI – a new perspective on benign breast disorders. *Br J Clin Pract* 1988; **42** (suppl 56): 1–9.
25. Smallwood JA, Roberts A, Guyer DP, Taylor I. The natural history of fibroadenomas. *Br J Clin Pract* 1988; **42** (suppl 56): 86–87.
26. Krainer WM, Rush BF. Mammary duct proliferation in the elderly: a histological study. *Cancer* 1973; **31**: 130–37.
27. Sloss PT, Bennett WA, Claydon OJ. Incidence in normal breast of features associated with chronic cystic mastitis. *Am J Pathol* 1957; **33**: 1181–98.
28. Page DL. Relationship between component parts of fibrocystic disease component parts of fibrocystic disease complex and breast cancer. *JNCI* 1978; **61**: 1055.

# 2

# Imaging in benign breast disease

P B GUYER

## Introduction

The objectives of imaging in clinically benign breast disease are both to confirm the clinical diagnosis, and to try and exclude unsuspected malignancy. Factors which hinder the attainment of these objectives are the background pattern of the breast on X-ray mammography, which, in its more severe forms, may hide serious disease,[1, 2] and the differentiation of small areas of calcification.

Attempts to improve the accuracy of breast imaging by overcoming the density problem have been made by using supplementary imaging techniques. Thermography was first used, but was dropped from the Breast Cancer Detection Demonstration Project (BCDDP) trial,[3] and, like scintigraphy and light scanning, is regarded as having insufficient specificity.[1, 3-8] A recent report,[9] however, has shown that modern light scanning has improved sensitivity, and this technique needs further careful evaluation.[10] Computed tomography has the dual disadvantages of a lengthy examination time and the use of irradiation,[5] and magnetic resonance imaging of the breast is still being developed.[4, 5, 11, 12] Only ultrasonography has proved to be generally clinically acceptable and sufficiently sensitive.[13-16] We have been using direct-contact static B-scan sonomammography for the past five years,[17-19] and the result of combining this with X-ray mammography has produced more accurate imaging diagnoses, as others have also reported.[20]

The fear of inducing breast cancer by repeated X-ray mammography[1, 21] has held back the widespread introduction of the examination but, with modern radiographic techniques, the radiation dose for a single exposure should be of the order of 1.2 mGy (0.12 rad); xerommamography gives a slightly higher dose. The theoretical risk of such doses is that one extra carcinoma would be produced per million women examined each year, and this is considered negligible in relation to the benefits of mammography.[1, 22-23] None the less, due to this and the problems caused by mammographic density in younger women, radiographic examination is normally reserved for patients aged 30 years or more, and ultrasonography can be used as the first examination in younger symptomatic patients.[1, 24-27]

## Background patterns in mammography

The presence of fat and glandular tissue in the breast leads to a mixture of radiolucent and radiodense areas on the mammogram, which range from total radiolucency (representing complete fat replacement) to near total radiodensity (reflecting dominance of grandular and stromal elements). There are mixed patterns of varying degrees between these two extremes. The fatty radiolucent breast is characteristic of most postmenopausal patients, and the radiodense breast is a feature of young patients, but there is considerable overlap with, in particular, occasional radiodensity in some postmenopausal breasts. An example of a typical mixed fatty/glandular pattern is shown in Fig. 2.1(a), and a normal sonomammogram in Fig. 2.1(b).

Three further background patterns are described – prominent ducts, ill defined rounded shadows, and more confluent areas of homogeneous density. Superadded to all these appearances there may be evidence of focal abnormalities – large or small areas of microcalcification, mass lesions, areas of focal density, or lucency, and disturbed trabeculation, all of which may occur alone or in various combinations.

Wolfe[28] initially described changes in the background pattern by drawing attention to ductal prominence. Mammograms without ductal prominence he labelled N 1, those with prominent ducts confined to the anterior quarter of the breast he labelled P1, and those with more extensive duct prominence, P2. His final classification was DY, which implied areas of confluent density which might be sufficient to obscure detail of the underlying parenchyma. Wellings and Wolfe[29] and Roebuck[30] added the description of larger (5–15 mm), ill defined rounded shadows as another variant of the background pattern (Fig. 2.2(a) and (b) ). These nodules tend to vary in size and distribution both within one breast and between the two breasts, resulting in some asymetry. Their definition is less than would be expected of cysts, which may also be present.

The third background variant consists of areas of homogenous density sometimes resulting in pronounced asymmetry between the two mammograms when they are compared (as they always should be) during interpretation (Fig. 2.3(a) and (b)). The importance of these patterns is controversial. Wolfe found a greater frequency of breast cancer in patients with P2 or DY patterns, and in the USA this can affect patient management.[29, 31, 32] Gravelle *et al*[33] agree with the risks of the P2 and DY pattern, but to a much lower factor than Wolfe suggested, and others[34, 35] doubt that there is any association. There are also suggestions of an association between the nodular pattern on mammography and breast cancer,[30] but this has not apparently been investigated by other workers.

a

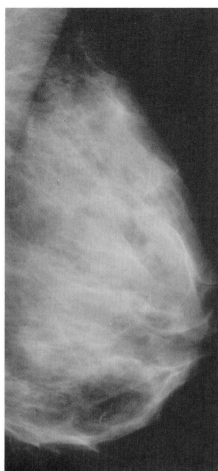

**Fig 2.1a** Normal X-ray mammogram – A fairly homogeneous distribution of density, interspread with more lucent areas representing fatty replacement.

**Fig 2.1b** Normal sonomammogram – the skin line is (a) a thin white line, beneath which is a fairly even, darker zone representing subcutaneous fat (b). There is a thin layer of retromammary fat (c), and in between there are regularly arranged intramammary fat lobules. Behind the breast lie the prepectoral fascia (d), pectoralis major (e), pleura (f), and lung.

b

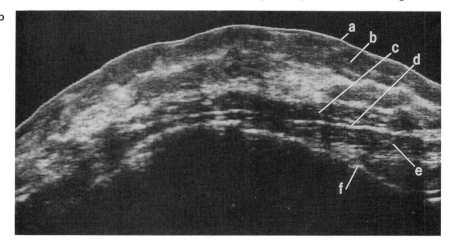

a

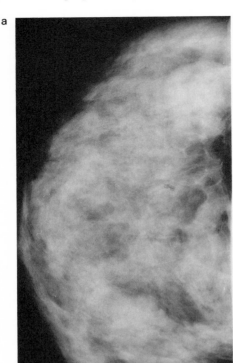

**Fig 2.2a** Diffusely nodular pattern – the breast parenchyma is uneven with poorly defined, rounded densities. These can be focal, rather than extensive, as in this illustration.

**Fig 2.2b** Sonomammogram in the same patient as fig. 2.2a. The central portion of the breast is replaced by a predominantly echo-bright pattern, indicating benign change in the breast.

b

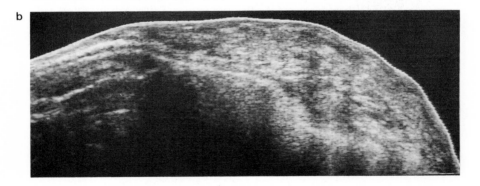

**Fig 2.3a** Asymmetrical density. There is a confluent density in the upper half of the right breast.

**Fig 2.3b** Sonomammogram in the patient illustrated in fig. 2.3(a) who complained of a right upper outer quadrant mass, so sonomammography was undertaken to elucidate the nature of the density. The central portion of the breast has been replaced by a mixture of bright and focal echo-poor areas. The appearances indicate benign (fibrocystic) changes and biopsy was averted. (Reproduced by kind permission of John Wiley and Sons).

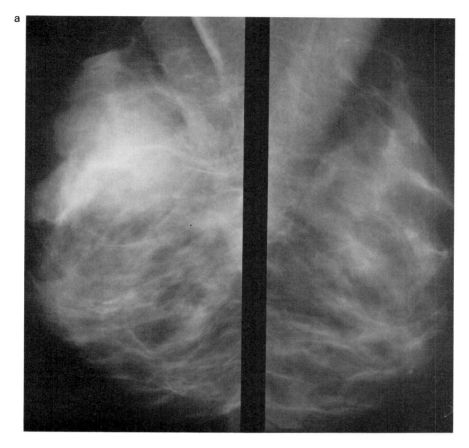

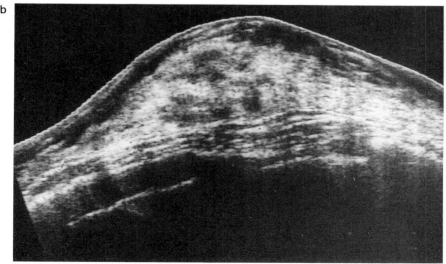

The ductal prominence described by Wolfe is now accepted to be caused by periductal fibrosis, and it is thought that the other patterns are produced by changes in the glands and stroma resulting from hormonal effects during growth, development, pregnancy, and involution.[36] They should therefore be regarded as being within the range of radiological normality and, because they are so frequent, they should be preferably not be labelled as diseases. This concept receives some support from the decrease in incidence of histological changes in postmenopausal women.[37]

Patients with these more diffuse benign changes may have a clinical lump, thickening, or nodularity, and may be found to have X-ray mammographic density within which it may be impossible to exclude a mass. Ultrasonography is indicated, because exclusion of a mass may make biopsy unnecessary; we have found that this use of ultrasonography reduces the benign biopsy rate by one third (Fig. 2.3(a) and (b) ).[19, 39]

There is clearly potential for considerable confusion if all these patterns are accepted, classified, and related to the risk of breast cancer. As they are a feature particularly of large screening series, they are of less relevance in the examination of symptomatic patients, and should therefore be used to indicate the need for careful examination of the mammograms to exclude a subclinical carcinoma. This is particularly so if there is a focal ductal prominence in one area of a breast, because this can be an indication of nearby malignancy. They should not be used by themselves to alter patient management – risk of cancer is more accurately indicated by histological and epidemiological factors.

The present terminology in benign breast processes urgently needs simplification and clarification and, until this is achieved, surgeons, pathologists, and radiologists need to agree locally on the terms to be used, and what they mean. Similar mammographic appearances may result from various histological appearances. In these there may be some overlap of microscopic changes, such as apocrine and epithelial hyperplasia, duct papillomatosis, and fibrocystic change.[10, 12, 38] With the possible exception of sclerosing adenosis, which may also show small microcalcification, it is generally not possible to identify these processes individually on mammograms, but in their various combinations they are considered responsible for the radiological changes of variable nodularity and density.[29]

## Localised lesions

### Microcalcifications

If these occur in sclerosing adenosis, they are usually rounded and discrete (Fig. 2.4(a) ), generally within the nodular areas, but sometimes visible in apparently normal breast tissue. Less commonly, they cluster (Figure 2.4(b) ), and then cause diagnostic problems because of overlap with malignant calcified areas, necessitating biopsy.[5, 40-43]

### *Microcysts*

These may be accompanied by microcalcifications which appear rounded and rather poorly defined on craniocaudad views, but give a 'tea cup' appearance on lateral projections, caused by sedimentation of the

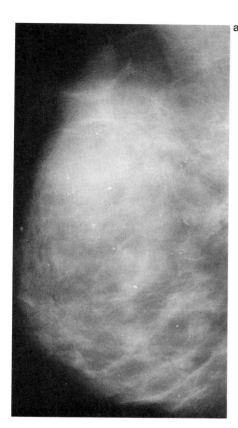

**Fig 2.4a** Sclerosing adenosis shown by a variable parenchymal pattern within which are discrete, mainly rounded, calcifications all of which are equally dense.

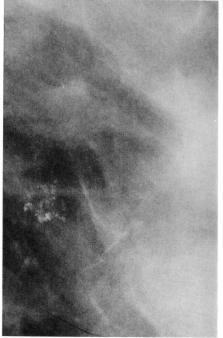

**Fig 2.4b** A less usual pattern in sclerosing adenosis, with clustered microcalcifications within which the individual calcifications look benign.

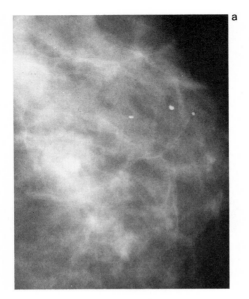

a

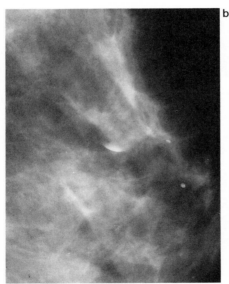

b

**Fig 2.5a&b** Microcysts shown as a poor marginated calcific density on the superior/inferior view, with layering of the calcium on the lateral view to form a crescent 'tea cup'.

calcified areas into the most dependent portion of the cyst (Fig. 2.5(a) and (b) ). Calcification in lobular hyperplasia may be similar.

*Epithelial hyperplasia and intraduct papillomatosis*

These two diseases cause small calcifications. In the latter condition, they tend to be confined to one breast segment and, if papillomatosis is florid, there may be multiple nodules in association with them. In both conditions the individual areas of calcification vary in size, and are generally rounded and poorly marginated, and with considerable variation in size within any one cluster (Fig. 2.6(a) and (b) ). When segmental, differentiation from multifocal or extensive intraduct carcinoma may be impossible except by examination of a biopsy specimen.

Unless calcifications are large, as in a fibroadenoma, they are unlikely to be shown by ultrasound scanning unless they are contained within a solid lesion. Thus ultrasonography will not detect the microcalcifications in sclerosis adenosis.

## Focal benign parenchymal masses

These share certain radiological features: they have well defined borders except where they lie against normal gland tissue; as they grow they may compress the surrounding breast tissue, the fat of which may produce a partial or complete thin lucent zone (halo) around the mass; and, with the exception of a galactocoele or an adenolipoma, they are all radio-dense, although the degree of density is rarely of diagnostic value. Thus many mammograms can only be reported as 'mass lesion, radiologically benign', and breast ultrasonography (sonomammography) may be needed to differentiate cystic from solid lesions.

*Fibroadenoma*

This is the commonest benign solid mass of the breast, being found most commonly during early childbearing ages, but known to occur with decreasing frequency throughout the reproductive period of life; they are uncommon after the menopause. They may enlarge considerably during pregnancy and lactation. Mammographically the mass is frequently lobulated and, in older patients, hyalinisation may occur, resulting in coarse calcifications which frequently lie towards the periphery of the mass. Fibroadenomas are multiple in 10–20% of patients (Fig. 2.7).[41] Since they occur in young patients, gland density may obscure the mass, and, in these, ultrasonography will be needed to reveal the lesion (Fig. 2.8(a) and (b) ).

Sonomammographic features of fibroadenoma are a well defined mass with an even internal echo pattern (Fig. 2.8(a) and (b) ). Two per cent of carcinomas are well defined radiologically, however, and have a surrounding halo, and these may also be sonographically well defined and evenly echogenic. In a series of 288 carcinomas[18] 16 were sonomammographically

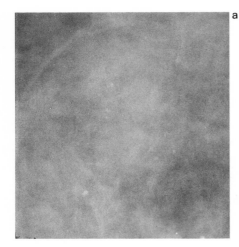

**Fig 2.6a** Epithelial hyperplasia – here calcifications vary in size, and are neither so sharp nor so dense as in sclerosing adenosis, although in individual cases differentiation might be difficult.

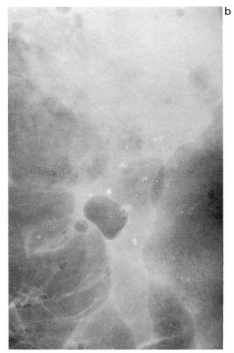

**Fig 2.6b** Excised specimen emphasising the variability in size of calcifications in epithelial hyperplasia.

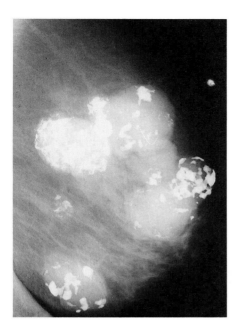

**Fig 2.7** Multiple calcified fibroadenomas showing good border definition; there is a partial halo effect with some, and the calcifications are typically coarse, tending to involve the periphery of the masses. (Reproduced by kind permission of John Wiley and Sons).

diagnosed as fibroadenomas because they were so well defined and had none of the characteristic ultrasound appearances of a breast cancer. Conversely, eight out of 89 proven fibroadenomas were labelled carcinoma on ultrasound scanning. If also clinically benign, the preoperative diagnosis will rest upon the result of fine needle aspiration.[44-46] Because of this imaging overlap, the radiological identification of a solid mass in a patient over the age of 30 years should lead to consideration of surgical excision.

Fibroadenomas may occasionally become very large, even occupying most of the breast. Although this is said to be commonest in older patients,[41] they are also seen in young females. Phyllodes tumour is variously considered to be a variant of fibroadenoma or a separate entity. In favour of the latter view is that approximately one in 14 of such tumours metastasise, or there may be local recurrence after excision.[10] Mammographically they are huge, well defined masses, occasionally containing coarse areas of calcification. Some of the tumours show fluid filled clefts on ultrasound scan (Fig. 2.9(a) and (b)).[19] Other benign solid masses, such as adenomas, fibromas, hamartomas, and neurofibromas, are likely to be diagnosed as fibroadenomas with both imaging techniques.

*Fibroadenolipoma*

This is, as the name implies, a mass of mixed fibrous, glandular, and fatty elements. With increasing use of mammography, these lesions are becoming more frequently recognised. Although they appear encapsulated (Fig. 2.10), this appearance is caused by compression of nearby trabeculae.[48]

a

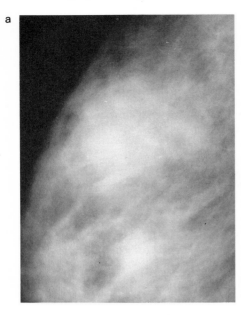

**Fig 2.8a**  Ill defined breast density in a patient complaining of a mass. There is a faint lucency anteriorly, suggesting that the mass may be benign.

**Fig 2.8b**  Sonomammogram in the same patient showing a mass which is well defined, especially posteriorly, with even echoes – a typical fibroadenoma.

b

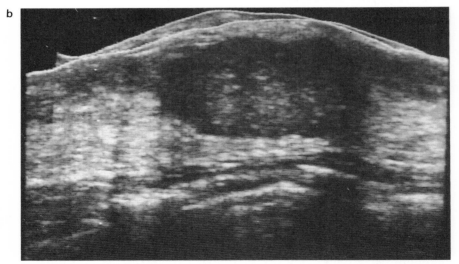

a

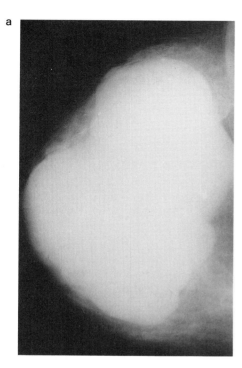

**Fig 2.9a** Phyllodes tumour – a huge, well defined, lobulated mass with a few coarse calcifications. (Reproduced by kind permission of John Wiley and Sons).

**Fig 2.9b** Ultrasound showing even echoes with the mass, but one or two small fluid clefts which are characteristic of phyllodes tumour, although not invariably found.

b

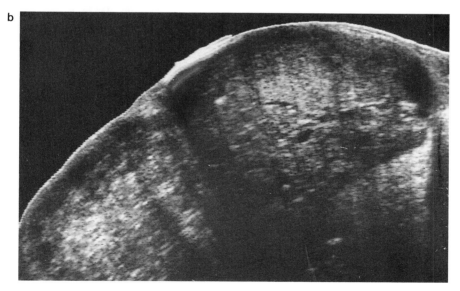

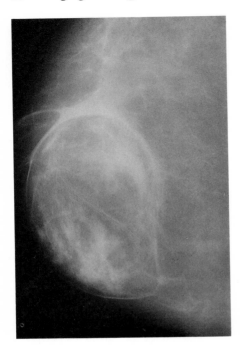

**Fig 2.10**   Fibroadendipoma – characteristic appearances of a well defined mass containing fatty and glandular elements.

Mammographically, the mass is a mixture of fatty and solid elements, and, on ultrasound scanning, is well defined and evenly echo containing. A lipoma is radiolucent, without the glandular elements.

There are some other small masses which may have distinctive features. A sebaceous cyst is well defined, but lies in the subcutaneous region on tangential views (Fig. 2.11(a)). Lymph nodes may occur either within or at the margin of the breast tissue. They are small, ovoid, and characteristically have a hilum and a relatively radiolucent centre (Fig. 2.11(b)). Vascular malformations are rarely seen in the breast (Fig. 2.11(c)), but look benign; ultrasonography may reveal the abnormal blood vessels. Cutaneous lesions are also well defined because of the air which surrounds them, as with cutaneous warts and nipple papillomas (Fig. 2.11(d)).

*Cysts*

Cysts are common; X-ray mammography will reveal more cysts than are suspected clinically, and ultrasonography will reveal still more, which occur in up to one third of patients aged 30–50 undergoing sonomammography.[19] As with fibroadenomas they are mammographically well defined, often with a surrounding halo of fat, but generally rounded rather than lobulated (Fig. 2.12(a)) They are frequently multiple and bilateral, and of varying size and visibility. If not under tension they may be ovoid. As with fibroadenomas they may be clearly shown on sonomammography; cysts

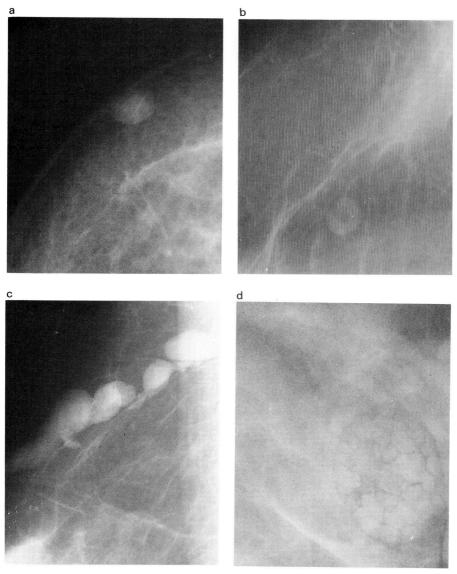

**Fig 2.11** Less frequent benign masses: (a) sebaceous cyst – diagnosed by the subcutaneous location; (b) lymph node with a characteristic central lucency and hilium; (c) a vascular malformation with a suggestive tortuous density; and (d) a cutaneous wart, with air in the crevices of the lesion.

a

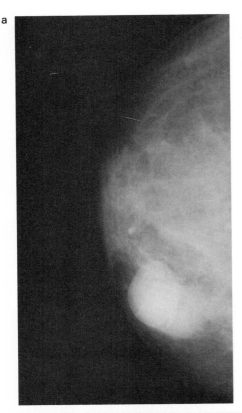

**Fig 2.12a** A cyst shown by a well defined sub areolar mass, with a partial fatty halo at its superior margin. Differentiation from other benign masses is not possible.

**Fig 2.12b** Sonomammogram confirming a cyst, but also revealing an intracystic papilloma.

b

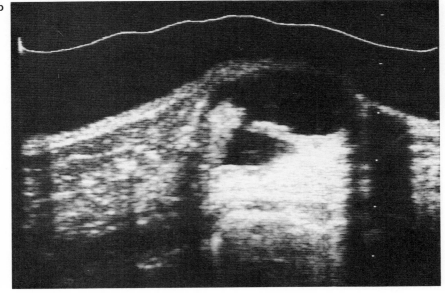

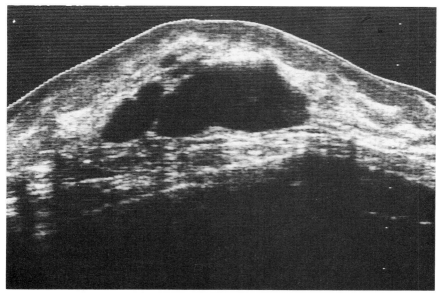

**Fig 2.12c** Typical appearances of cysts on ultrasound, with well defined echo free masses. The ovoid shapes indicate that they are not under tension.

may also be well shown by ultrasonography after breast augmentation. On ultrasound scanning some cysts may have echogenic contents, raising the possibility of a solid, rather than cystic, lesion; this can be resolved by ultrasound guided aspiration at the time of the examination. Intracystic papillomas will resemble a cyst on X-ray mammography, and the papilloma will only be shown by ultrasonography (Fig. 2.12(b)) or pneumocystography. If haemorrhage occurs into the cyst, a clue to the fact that this is not a straightforward cyst might be considerable density of the mass.[42] In the author's experience, intracystic carcinoma is rare[51] – only one case has been seen locally.[49] Rarely cysts develop a rim of calcification.

The ultrasonographic sensitivity for cysts is 98%, so that for patients with previously known cystic disease, breast ultrasound scanning could be undertaken as the first examination[25, 50] with X-ray mammography to follow if there is a dubious mass on the ultrasound scan (Fig. 2.12(c)).

## Focal stromal lesions

These represent a reaction of the breast to a stimulus which may be infective or traumatic. The lesions are unilateral, and produce a palpable abnormality of variable size with pain (at least initially) of variable intensity. They share some common X-ray features, such as an ill defined density or mass, a tissue response by the breast in the form of oedema or marginal striations, and variable skin thickening. Without knowledge of the clinical history, the wrong mammographic diagnosis is easily reached as some of these are indistinguishable from carcinoma.

*Plasma cell mastitis*

This is a stromal inflammatory response to the escape of infected contents from the ducts (Fig. 2.13(a) and (b) ). It is, therefore, commonly seen in the subareolar region, but may occur at other sites. There is a unilateral or asymmetrical breast density which is poorly defined because of the oedema and increased vascularity, and with irregular marginal striations caused by lymphatic engorgement or a fibrotic response. Well defined ductal calcifications of the linear and ring type may give a clue to the underlying ductal disease. Sonomammography reveals an ill defined density with attenuation deep to it, and an area of superficial bright echoes which may interrupt the subcutaneous fat (Fig. 2.13(b) ). There is a pronounced degree of overlap here with fat necrosis and carcinoma.[52, 53]

*Haematoma*

Haematoma may be the result of external injury, in which case, when acute, it resembles fat necrosis. It may also be caused by the use of anticoagulants, or a low platelet count. With biopsy and surgery of the breast, however, haematomas may be deeply placed and more focal (Fig. 2.14(a) ), closely similar to the chronic stage of fat necrosis. Ultrasound scan at this time will show a fairly well defined mass, clearly containing some fluid, as well as internal echoes due to debris (Fig. 2.14(b) ).

*Fat necrosis*

Fat necrosis, for all practical purposes, is radiologically indentical with plasma cell mastitis in the acute phases, but the clue to the diagnosis lies in the history, and, because of the injury, the skin tends to be thickened. Chronic changes may show a focal density with a spiculated margin (Fig. 2.14(d) ), strongly suggestive of carcinoma. With healing, lipid cysts may form, with ring calcification in their walls (Fig. 2.15).[54]

*Abscess*

An abscess is normally clinically apparent and mammography is unlikely to be tolerated in the early stages because of pain, but when it is slow to resolve an ill defined density is shown mammographically; this is occasionally well defined in places due to compression of adjacent fat. Ultrasonography shows a less well defined cavity than with the haematoma, but still containing fluid and solid areas (Fig. 2.14(c)). With both haematoma and abscess, the diagnosis can be confirmed by needle aspiration; if this fails, then ultrasound guided aspiration is likely to succeed.

*Sclerosing adenosis*

This may present as a breast lump,[55] but this is uncommon. The mammographic appearances are likely to resemble carcinoma with a

a

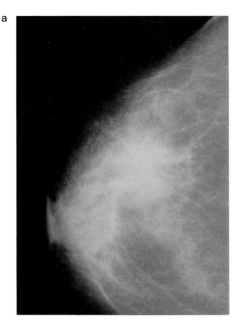

**Fig 2.13a** Plasma cell mastitis shown by an ill defined density that is centrally placed, with some marginal striations. Fat necrosis, early haematoma, and even carcinoma may appear similar – the history is critical. (Reproduced by kind permission of John Wiley and Sons).

**Fig 2.13b** Sonomammogram in the patient illustrated in fig. 2.13(a) showing extensive central shadowing (attenuation) with superficial, bright echoes. Absence of a tumour makes the presence of carcinoma less likely but fat necrosis is indistinguishable.

b

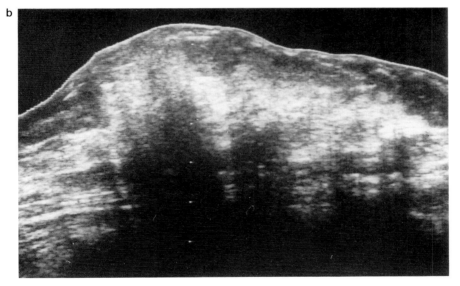

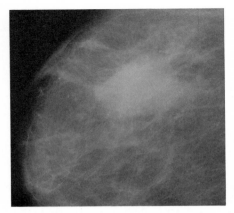

**Fig 2.14a** Haematoma resulting from biopsy. There is a suspiciously striated mass with tethering and skin thickening; without the history carcinoma would be diagnosed.

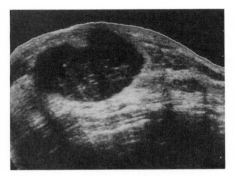

**Fig 2.14b** Circumscribed haematoma shown by ultrasound, with sharp definition of the border and multiple internal echoes. The differentiation from a cyst with echo containing fluid could be made by aspiration during the ultrasound examination.

suspiciously stellate density containing calcifications; the differentiation is likely to require biopsy.[53]

*Radial scar*

Radial scar is a diagnosis which has attracted much attention in recent years, and has been given a variety of histological labels, such as sclerosing papillary proliferations, benign sclerosing ductal proliferations, infiltrative epitheliosis, and indurative mastopathy.[56] Although it was originally thought to be premalignant, this has now been discounted[57] and it is considered to be part of the spectrum of benign breast change which includes

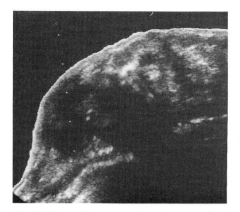

**Fig 2.14c** Abscess, showing poor border definition to an area containing both fluid and solid components. Attempted aspiration in the out-patient clinic failed, but under ultrasound guidance the fluid containing areas were aspirated, revealing pus.

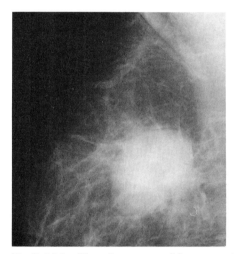

**Fig 2.14d** Chronic stages of fat necrosis, showing a spiculated mass mimicking carcinoma.

fibrocystic disease and sclerosing adenosis.[58] Azzopardi[38] commented on the wide range and overlapping histological appearances which histologically may mimic carcinoma, and the overlap with malignancy may also occur mammographically.[42] The radiological appearances are of fine striae of variable length radiating to a nidus with a lucent centre (Fig. 2.16). The striae may be separated by fatty lucencies. None the less, the similarity to carcinoma is such that biopsy is probably unavoidable in order to establish the diagnosis.[59]

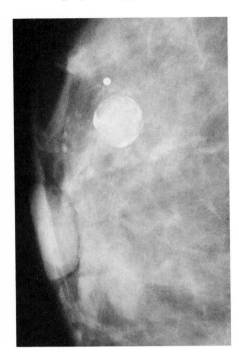

**Fig 2.15** A lipid cyst following trauma. The fairly extensive rim calcification makes this appear dense, whereas without the calcification it would appear radio lucent.

## Silicone injections

Silicone injections used to be used for breast augmentation, but the material promotes a fibrotic response, producing a characteristic X-ray appearance (Fig. 2.17) of diffuse poorly defined densities, and trabecular disturbances resulting from the fibrotic response.

## Ductal abnormalities

Ductal calcification is commonly seen, and takes two forms (Fig. 2.18): parallel calcified areas in the duct walls which are circular when seen in cross section, and linear intraductal calcified areas, which tend to have smooth regular margins and which occasionally branch.[12] There is some debate as to whether these linear calcifications lie within or alongside the inflamed ducts.[40] They result from ductal dilatation and inflammation, and thus may be a feature of plasma cell mastitis.

## Duct ectasia

Duct ectasia is shown by prominent tubular shadows, particularly in the subareolar region (Fig. 2.19). When associated with periductal inflammation it may result in nipple retraction,[60] although the same authors comment that it is not possible to differentiate periductal shadowing from duct dilatation

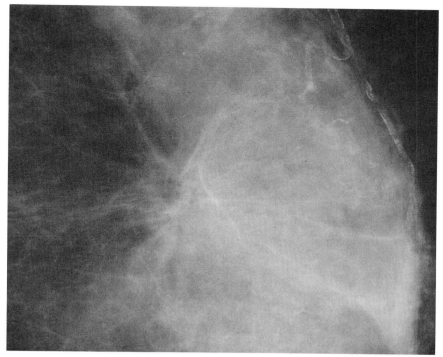

**Fig 2.16**   A radial scar shown by striae radiating from a central point within which there is a lucent area. Differentiation from carcinomas will normally require biopsy. (Note the vascular calcification superficially.)

unless the latter has a high lipid content, in which case the contents are radio-lucent. Such dilatation of the duct system deep in the breast may result in galactocoeles (Fig. 2.20).[61] Dilatation of a solitary duct may be the only clue to a small intraduct papilloma or carcinoma, and needs to be regarded with considerable suspicion.

Where there is nipple discharge, and particularly if it is bloodstained, ductography can be used. It may define duct estasia more accurately,[62] and can identify intraduct papillomas, although inspissated secretions can cause diagnostic problems. Breast cysts can be opacified by ductography, and occasionally carcinomas may be detected by duct distortion, narrowing, and obstruction.[63] The technique is safe, and may help with preoperative localisation of suspected ductal pathology.

## The male breast

In men the breast contains few gland elements and it is therefore normally radiolucent, with just a few strands representing residual ducts or fibrous stroma. Breast enlargement can be due to obesity, gynaecomastia, or

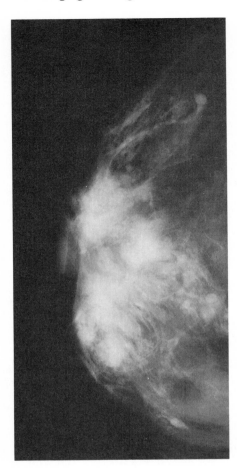

**Fig 2.17** Silicone injection for breast augmentation resulting in diffuse, ill defined densities and widespread trabecular disturbance.

neoplasia; with obesity, there is merely an excess of fat. In gynaecomastia there is a proliferation of stromal and glandular elements,[12, 64, 65] resulting mammographically in a triangular or rounded subareolar density if acute, and dendritic density if longstanding.[66] Gynaecomastia is most commonly seen in association with hormonal therapy for prostate cancer, but may also occur with a variety of drugs including digitalis, thiazides, spironolactone, and addictive drugs.[65] It also occurs in general medical conditions such as cirrhosis, renal failure with dialysis, and adrenal and testicular tumours. Occasionally papillomas associated with gynaecomastia may give rise to a bloodstained discharge.

Carcinoma of the male breast is rare, representing less than 1% of all breast cancers. It does not differ mammographically from cancer of the female breast, except that small areas of calcification are less common.[65] Cysts are rare in the male breast.[67]

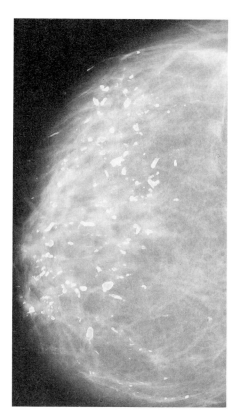

Fig 2.18 Ductal wall calcifications appearing as parallel linear densities when the duct is seen longitudinally, and as circular densities in cross section. There are also fine single linear calcifications indicating intra-luminal calcifications.

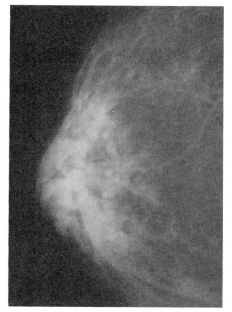

Fig 2.19 Duct ectasia shown by tortuous tubular shadows deep to the nipple.

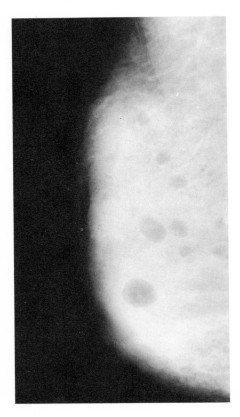

**Fig 2.20** Galactocoeles shown as radio lucent rounded shadows (due to their lipid contents) contrasted against the dominant density of the breast glandular tissue.

## Conclusions

While the debate continues about the background parenchymal pattern of the breast, in symptomatic patients the detection of a risk pattern should ensure a particularly careful examination of the mammograms. Most of the observed patterns represent hormonal changes or variations of normal, and should be regarded as benign breast changes rather than benign breast disease.

In patients with X-ray dense breasts, X-ray mammography should be supplemented by sonomammography, particularly if there is an obvious mass. Not only will this increase the information gained and give greater diagnostic confidence, but it can also detect carcinoma in clinically benign disease. It is valuable in the investigation of a radiologically indeterminate mass. By excluding a focal mass, it can help to reduce the need for surgery. Suspected cysts which resist aspiration in the outpatient clinic should undergo ultrasound examination with a view to ultrasound guided aspiration, and this can also be used for the aspiration of haematomas and abscesses. Additional indications for sonomammography rather than X-ray mammography are symptoms in a patient under 30 years of age, severe physical disability, severe mastalgia, and following augmentation. It should also be used for breast symptoms in pregnancy.

# References

1. Kopans DB, Meyer JE, Sadowsky N. Breast imaging. *N Engl J Med* 1984; **310**: 960–67.
2. Cahill DJ, Boulter PS, Gibbs NM, Price JL. Features of mammographically negative breast tumours. *Br J Surg* 1981; **68**: 882–89.
3. Martin JE. Breast imaging techniques. *Radiol Clin North Am* 1983; **21**: 149–53.
4. Sickles EA. Breast imaging. *Diagn Imag Clin Med* 1985; **54**: 118–25.
5. Homer MJ. Breast imaging: pitfalls, controversies, and some practical thoughts. *Radiol Clin North Am* 1985; **23**: 459–72.
6. Den Outer AJ, Parwels EKJ, Zwaveling A, *et al.* Breast scintigraphy for the detection of malignant disease. *Br J Surg* 1986; **73**: 813–14.
7. Monsees B, Destrouet JM, Gersell D. Light scan evaluation of impalpable breast lesions. *AJR* 1987; **163**: 467–70.
8. Milbraith JR. Thermography. In: Bassett LW, Gold RH. (Eds) *Breast Cancer Detection*. New York, Grune & Stratton Inc, 1987, pp. 145–52.
9. Dowle S, Caseldine J, Tew J, *et al.* An evaluation of transmission spectography in the diagnosis of symptomatic breast lesions. *Clin Radiol.* 1985; **38**: 375–77.
10. D'Orsi CJ, Feldhaus L, Sonnerfeld M. Unusual lesions of the breast. *Radiol Clin North Am* 1983; **21**: 67–80.
11. Dash N, Lupetin AR, Dattner RH, *et al.* MRI in the diagnosis of breast disease. *AJR* 1986; **146**: 119–25.
12. Bassett LW, Gold RH, Cove HC. Mammographic spectrum of traumatic fat necrosis. *AJR* 1978; **130**: 119–22.
13. Jellins J, Reeve TS. Breast echography compared with xerography. *Ultrasound in Medicine* 1978; **4**: 313–18.
14. Kelly-Fry E. Breast imaging – In: Sabanga RE. (Ed) *Diagnostic Ultrasound in Obstetrics and Gynaecology*. Hagerstown, Harper and Row, 1980, pp. 327–50.
15. Cole–Beuglet C, Kurtz AB, Rubin CS, Goldberg BB. Ultrasound mammography. *Radiol Clin North Am* 1980; **18**: 133–43.
16. McSweeney MB, Murphy CH. Whole breast sonography. *Radiol Clin North Am* 1985; **23**: 157–67.
17. Guyer PB, Dewbury KC. Ultrasound of the breast in the symptomatic X-ray dense breast. *Clin Radiol* 1985; **36**: 69–76.
18. Guyer PB, Dewbury KC, Warwick D, *et al.* Direct-contact B-scan ultrasound in the diagnosis of solid breast masses. *Clin Radiol* 1986; **37**: 451–58.
19. Guyer PB, Dewbury KC. *Sonomammography: an Atlas of Comparative Breast Ultrasound* Chichester, John Wiley & Sons Ltd., 1987.
20. Fleischer AC, Muhletar CA, Reynolds VH, *et al.* Palpable breast masses: evaluation by high-frequency hand-held real-time sonography and xero-mammography. *Radiology* 1983; **148**: 813–17.
21. Bailar J. Mammography: a contrary view. *Ann Intern Med* 1976; **84**: 77–83.
22. Feig S. Radiation risk from mammography. *AJR* 1984; **143**: 469–75.
23. Strax P. Imaging of the breast. *Surg Clin North Am* 1984; **64**: 1063–72.
24. Harper P, Kelly-Fry E. Ultrasound visualisation of the breast in symptomatic patients. *Radiology* 1980; **137**: 465–69.
25. Croll J, Kotevich J, Tabrett M. The diagnosis of benign disease and the exclusion of malignancy in patients with breast symptoms. *Seminars in Ultrasound* 1982; **3**: 38–50.

26. Egan RL, Egan KL. Detection of breast cancer, *AJR* 1984; **143**: 493–97.
27. Walsh P, Baddesley H, Timms H, Furnival CM. An assessment of ultrasound mammography as an additional investigation for the diagnosis of breast disease. *Br J Radiol* 1985; **58**: 115–19.
28. Wolfe JN. A study of breast parenchyma by mammography in the normal woman and those with benign and malignant disease. *Radiology* 1976; **89**: 201–5.
29. Wellings SR, Wolfe JN. Correlative studies of the histological and radiographic appearances of the breast parenchyma. *Radiology* 1978; **129**: 299–306.
30. Roebuck EJ. The importance of mammographic parenchymal pattern. *Br J Radiol* 1982; **55**: 387–98.
31. Wolfe JN. Breast patterns as an index of the risk for developing breast cancer. *AJR* 1976; **126**: 1130–39.
32. Wolfe JN. Risk of developing breast cancer determined by mammography. (Eds) In: *Prog Clin. Biol. Res.* 1977; **12**: 223–238
33. Gravelle IH, Bulstrode JC, Bulbrook RD *et al*. A prospective study of mammographic parenchymal patterns and risk of breast cancer. *B J Radiol* 1986; **59**: 487–91.
34. Moskowitz M, Gartside P, McLaughlin C. Mammographic markers for high-risk benign breast disease and incident cancer. *Radiology* 1980; **134**: 293–95.
35. Verbeck ALM, Hendricks JHCL, Peeters PHM, Sturmans F. Mammographic patterns and the risk of breast cancer. *Lancet* 1984; **i**: 591–93.
36. Hughes LE, Mansell, RE, Webster DJ. Aberrations of normal development and involution (ANDI): a new perspective and pathogenesis and nomenclature of benign breast disease. *Lancet* 1987; **ii**: 1316–19.
37. Devitt JE. Benign disorders of the breast in older women. *Surg Gynecol Obstet* 1986; **162**: 340–42.
38. Azzopardi JG. Problems in breast pathology. In: Bennington JL (Consultant Ed): *Major Problems in Pathology*, vol. II, Philadelphia 1979. London, WB Saunders & Co., 1979, pp. 168–74.
39. McSweeney MB, Egan RL. Automated breast sonography: comparison with other modalities – ultrasonic examination of the breast. In: *Ultrasonic Examination of the Breast* Ed. Jellins J, Kobayashi T. Chichester, John Wiley & Sons Ltd., 1983, pp. 325–33.
40. Muir BB, Lamb J, Anderson TJ, Kirkpatrick AE. Microcalcification and its relationship to cancer of the breast, *Clin Radiol* 1983; **34**: 193–200.
41. Paulus DD. Benign disease of the breast. *Radiol Clin North Am* 1983; **21**: 27–50.
42. Tabar L, Dean PB. In: Fronimhold W, Thurn P. (Eds) *Teaching Atlas of Mammography*. Stuttgart, George Thieme Verlag, 1983, pp. 119–29.
43. Hansell DM, Cooke JC, Parsons CA, *et al*. A quantitative analysis of the spatial relationship of grouped microcalcifications. *Br J Radiol* 1988; **61**: 21–5.
44. Smallwood J, Khong Y, Boyd A, *et al*. An assessment of a scoring scheme for the pre-operative diagnosis of breast lumps. *Ann R Coll Surg Engl* 1984; **66**: 267–69.
45. Smallwood J, Herbert A, Guyer P, Taylor I. Accuracy of aspiration cytology in the diagnosis of breast disease. *Br J Surg* 1985; **72**: 841–43.
46. Smallwood J, Guyer PB, Dewbury KC, *et al*. The accuracy of ultrasound in the diagnosis of breast disease. *Ann R Coll Surg Engl* 1986; **68**: 19–22.
47. McDevitt RW, Farrow JH, Stewart FW. Breast carcinoma arising in a solitary fibroadenoma. *Surg Gynecol Obstet* 1967; **125**: 572–76.
48. Crothers JG, Butler NF, Fortt RW, Gravelle IH. Fibro-adenolipoma of the breast. *Br J Radiol* 1985; **58**: 191–202.
49. Reuter K, D'Orsi CJ, Reale F. Intracystic carcinoma of the breast. *Radiology* 1984; **153**: 233–34.

50. Rosner D, Blaird D. What ultrasound can tell that clinical examination and X-Ray cannot. *J Surg Oncol* 1985; **28**: 308–13.
51. Tabar L, Dean PB. Interventional radiological procedures in the investigation of lesions of the breast. *Radiol Clin North Am* 1981; **17**: 607–21.
52. Haagensen CD. Mammary duct ectasia; a disease that may mimic carcinoma. *Cancer* 1951; **4**: 749–61.
53. Gold RH, Montgomery CK, Rambo ON. Significance of margination of benign and malignant infiltrative mammary lesions. *AJR* 1973; **118**: 881–94.
54. Bassett LW, Gold RH, Cove HC. Mammographic spectrum of traumatic fat necrosis. *AJR* 1978; **130**: 119–112.
55. Nielsen NSM, Nielsen BB. Mammographic features of sclerosing adenosis presenting as a tumour. *Clin Radiol* 1986; **37**: 371–73.
56. Sloane JP, Trott PA. *Biopsy Pathology of the Breast.* London, Chapman Hall, pp. 87–91.
57. Nielsen M, Jensen J, Andersen JA. An autopsy study of radial scar in the female breast. *Histopathology* 1985; **9**: 287–95.
58. Anderson JA, Gram JB. Radial scar in the female breast. *Cancer* 1984; **53**: 2557–60.
59. Price JL, Thomas BA, Gibbs NM. The mammographic features of infiltrating epitheliosis. *Clin Radiol* 1983; **34**: 433–35.
60. Rees BI, Gravelle IH, Hughes LE. Nipple retraction in duct ectasia. *Br J Surg* 1977; **64**: 577–80.
61. Gomez A, Mata JM, Donaso L, Rans A. Galactocele: three distinctive radiographic appearances. *Radiology* 1986; **158**: 43–4.
62. Threatt B. Ductography. In: Bassett LW, Gold Rh. (Eds) *Breast Cancer Detection.* New York, Grune & Stratton Inc, 1987, pp. 119–29.
63. Tabar L, Dean PB, Pentek Z. Galactography: the diagnostic procedure of choice for nipple discharge. *AJR* 1983; **149**: 31–8.
64. Kapdi CC, Parekh NJ. The male breast. *Radiol Clin North Am* 1983; **21**: 137–48.
65. Dershaw DD. Male mammography. *AJR* 1986; **146**: 127–31.
66. Michels LG, Gold RH, Arndt RD. Radiography of gynaecomastia and other disorders of the male breast. *Radiology* 1977; **122**: 117–22.
67. Weshler Z, Sulkes A. Contrast mammography and the diagnosis of male breast cysts. *Clin Radiol* 1980; **31**: 341–43.

# 3

# Mastalgia

P E PREECE

## Definiton and incidence

The term mastalgia means 'breast pain'; it is a symptom, not a disease. To emphasise this, the word 'mastalgia' is used in preference to the word 'mastodynia', a word which also literally means breast pain, but which has been used on occasions in the past to imply particular histopathological entities.[1, 2] A study of young women in Scottish hospitals in 1965 showed that 40% had some premenstrual mastalgia.[3] The frequency with which patients present with this symptom in general practice in a Southern English city was reported by Nichols in 1980 as 52% of all breast complaints.[4] Obviously the symptom is common. Is it important? If so, to whom and in what circumstances? To answer these questions it is necessary to have a classification and a differential diagnosis of mastalgia.

## Classification

Mastalgia is best subclassified as non-breast mastalgia, cyclical mastalgia, and non-cyclical mastalgia.

### Non-breast mastalgia

Conditions which have no association either with the breast or the chest wall sometimes cause mastalgia.

### Cyclical mastalgia

Any sensation which is experienced by 40% of the population might be regarded as normal or physiological. Sensation of heightened awareness, discomfort, fullness, and heaviness in the breasts during the three to seven days which precede each mensis and which often disappear suddenly with the commencement of the menstrual flow should be regarded as physiological. For some women 'physiological' cyclical mastalgia becomes so intense that relief of symptoms is requested. The term 'cyclical pronounced' is useful to describe this. The other commonly encountered variation of physiological mastalgia for which relief is sought is 'cyclical prolonged' when, rather than the breast symptoms being present for just a few days late in each menstrual cycle, they recommence almost as soon as the menstrual flow stops and gain intensity until the beginning of the next mensis. For some women cyclical prolonged mastalgia can be present for from three quarters to the whole of each menstrual cycle, thereby interfering with normal living.

## Non-cyclical mastalgia

Non-cyclical mastalgia is breast pain with a time pattern that is not associated with cyclical ovarian function. It may be continuous, but usually has a random time pattern.

# Differential diagnosis

Possible causes for breast pain that arise outside the breast are best considered before local causes. Non-breast mastalgia can be caused by angina, cholelithiasis, degenerative disorders such as cervical spondylosis, hiatus hernia, nerve entrapment syndromes as in carpal tunnel or cervical rib, oesophageal lesions particularly achalasia, pleurisy from pneumonia, or pulmonary tuberculosis.

Cyclical mastalgia, whether pronounced or prolonged, is inextricably linked with the function of the pituitary ovarian axis. It might therefore be thought of as systemic in origin.

Non-cyclical mastalgia is associated with a wide range of apparently unrelated events and conditions. These are usually local rather than systemic – that is, their causes are located either in the breast or chest wall. Particular benign breast disorders which are strongly associated with non-cyclical mastalgia are duct ectasia, fat necrosis, and sclerosing adenosis. The chest wall disorder commonly called Tietze's syndrome, where one or more of the costal cartilages posterior to the breast is enlarged, painful, and tender, often presents as non-cyclical mastalgia.[5]

## Duct ectasia

Non-cyclical mastalgia attributable to duct ectasia is distinctive in a number of respects (Table 3.1). Mammograms in these patients often show features pointing to the presence of duct ectasia, such as prominent ducts or clusters of areas of coarse calcification.[6, 7]

## Fat necrosis

Fat necrosis in the breast is usually the result of trauma caused by either

**Table 3.1**   Distinctive clinical features of non-cyclical mastalgia associated with duct ectasia

- Burning pain
- Exacerbated by cold
- Site precisely located
- Often subareolar or upper inner quadrant
- Tender to touch

accidental injury or compression by an abscess or incision for biopsy. Non-cyclical mastalgia often occurs at the sites of such injuries, in many cases months or years after the originating event. No doubt scarring occurs in the interim and usually this can be detected either clinically, or radiologically, or both. The reason why these scars become a locus of pain is not apparent. A notable feature of non-cyclical mastalgia after trauma is that it is much more often associated with radial scars – that is, scars of incisions made across Langer's lines of election rather than parallel to, or in, them. It is also more likely to follow biopsies which were complicated by haematomata.

**Sclerosing adenosis**

Sclerosing adenosis associated with localised non-cyclical mastalgia may be easier to understand than the links between pain and duct ectasia or fat necrosis. Sclerosing adenosis is a well recognised histopathological entity consisting of proliferative glandular epithelium in which fibrosis distorts the normal pattern of the lobule.[8-10] Proliferating epithelial cells in this condition have been described as invading both nerves and blood vessels.[11, 12] It is tempting to speculate that either the epithelial proliferation or the pronounced fibrosis causes the pain which has been reported as a symptom in 50% of a series of 43 sequential cases with this histopathological diagnosis.[13] The finding of sclerosing adenosis by the histopathologist can be anticipated in patients with well localised non-cyclical mastalgia whose mammograms show a collection of small areas of calcification in the breast at the site of pain.

Occasionally non-cyclical mastalgia is associated with mammary malignancy. It is ironical that breast cancers so rarely cause pain in their early, localised stage of development. The question of whether pain is really a symptom of some early breast cancers (or whether these are found by chance when investigations are performed for mastalgia) has been and remains controversial. A number of authors have reported that mastalgia can be a symptom of operable breast cancer.[14-18] Evidence to support the opposite view, however, has been published.[19-22] In a four year series of 240 operable breast cancers in patients whose symptoms were recorded prospectively at presentation (before examination and investigation),[18] mastalgia corresponding to the site of the tumour had been experienced by 36, whose ages ranged from 31 to 77 years. It was the sole presenting symptom in 17, of which five were impalpable $T_0$ lesions. Whether cancer is actually locally painful or not, pain in a breast can result in the detection of this disease, often at an early stage. A remarkably high proportion, (namely six, 17%) of the 36 cancer patients complaining of breast pain had invasive lobular carcinoma as their final diagnosis. This suggests that lobular carcinoma has a special propensity to cause pain. This histopathological type of breast cancer has been shown to be particularly difficult to diagnose by cryostat histology[16] and on mammograms.[23] Awareness that it may cause mastalgia could result in its being diagnosed earlier.

## Anatomy, physiology, and natural history of mastalgia

### Anatomy

The sensory nerve supply of the skin over the breasts is derived from the anterior and middle branches of the second, third, fourth, and fifth intercostal nerves and the upper borders are supplied by the supraclavicular branches of the cervical plexus.[24] The phenomenon of 'referred' pain can result in, first, pain originating from outside the breasts being experienced in those organs, for example from irritation of a cervical nerve root by spondylosis; secondly, pain originating within the breast may radiate to other sites which receive their sensory innervation from the same nerve roots as the breast, for example, the axilla and the upper medial part of the arm.

### Physiology

The sex hormone changes of the menstrual cycle are implicitly linked with cyclical mastalgia. The particular hormones that are altered and the way that this occurs are not known, despite our ability to measure blood concentrations of such hormones as oestrogen and progesterone, luteinising hormone, and follicle stimulating hormone. To date the most convincing theories point to possible alterations in prolactin metabolism in women who have troublesome cyclical mastalgia. Such women, when tested with prolactin secretion provocation tests, mounted much higher peak prolactin concentrations than symptom-free age matched controls.[25] This phenomenon has been correlated with both high nocturnal secretion of prolactin[26] and with the achievement of a good response to endocrine treatment of the mastalgia.[27]

### Natural history

Five to 10 year follow up of premenopausal patients with mastalgia managed 'conservatively' – that is by reassurance but without medication or surgery – showed that the majority with unilateral pain were free of this within two or three years. Half of patients with bilateral mastalgia still experienced this three to four years after they presented, and a third of such women still had symptoms at eight years.[28] The menopause, however, brought relief to the majority, which was also found in a more recent 10 year prospective study of 200 mastalgia sufferers, many of whom were treated medically.[29]

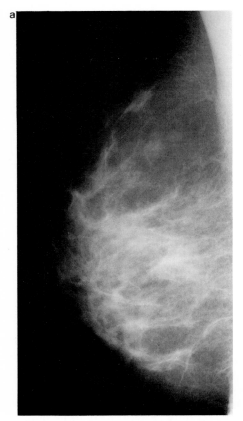

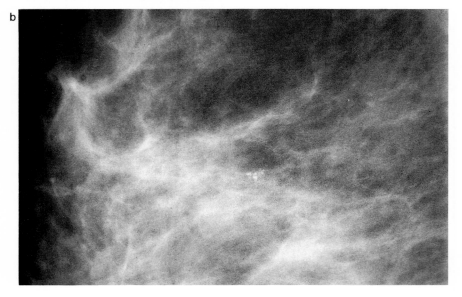

**Fig 3.1** Mammogram with a small collection of areas of calcification at a site from which biopsy showed a sclerosing adenosis; (a) whole mammogram, and (b) magnified segment.

## Investigation

The initial investigation of women complaining of breast pain should be those appropriate to any patient of comparable age experiencing any locoregional breast symptoms. For all there will be clinical examination. For those with lumps, fine needle aspiration cytology is most valuable. Mammograms can be helpful in those in whom it is likely that there will be sufficiently good radiolucency of the breasts to yield information. In general, for most British breast clinics, this would mean no mammograms for patients less than 30 years old. These investigations are intended primarily to exclude malignant disease. They may yield positive information indicating the aetiology of the mastalgia (for example, prominent mammary ducts may indicate the presence of duct ectasia). Ultrasonography may also add further information. The single most useful test for patients with mastalgia is a 'breast pain chart' (Fig. 3.2). This is a calendar card on which the patient may record the frequency and the severity of her breast pain.[30] A parallel line of boxes to record events of the menstrual cycle enables easy recognition of any pattern the breast pain has in relation to the menses. Such a chart also provides a quantitative way of measuring responses to treatment.

## Treatment

### Conservative treatment

Clinicians, particularly surgeons, have regarded the complaint of mastalgia as an expression of neurosis, and the fact that patients with pain in the breast

BREAST PAIN - DAILY PAIN CHART

Shade in each box on the day you get any breast pain

For example:-

Severe pain

Mild pain

• No pain

If you get breast pain on the fifth day of the month then shade in the square under No. 5. Please note the day your period starts each month with the letter 'P'.

DATE

| MONTH | 1 | 2 | 3 | 4 | 5 | 6 | 7 | 8 | 9 | 10 | 11 | 12 | 13 | 14 | 15 | 16 | 17 | 18 | 19 | 20 | 21 | 22 | 23 | 24 | 25 | 26 | 27 | 28 | 29 | 30 | 31 |
|---|---|---|---|---|---|---|---|---|---|---|---|---|---|---|---|---|---|---|---|---|---|---|---|---|---|---|---|---|---|---|---|
| | | | | | | | | | | | | | | | | | | | | | | | | | | | | | | | |
| | | | | | | | | | | | | | | | | | | | | | | | | | | | | | | | |
| | | | | | | | | | | | | | | | | | | | | | | | | | | | | | | | |
| | | | | | | | | | | | | | | | | | | | | | | | | | | | | | | | |
| | | | | | | | | | | | | | | | | | | | | | | | | | | | | | | | |
| | | | | | | | | | | | | | | | | | | | | | | | | | | | | | | | |

Please bring this card with you on each visit.

**Fig 3.2** Daily breast pain chart.

are often anxious has reinforced this. They have been called such things as hypochondriacal, or irritable, or nervous. Reassurance has long been recognised as a necessary part of management. Theodor Billroth wrote that: 'Friendly advice, reassurance and the banishment of suspicion and fear of dread disease is of great importance'.[14] Geschickter defined three principles for managing the complaint: 'Exclude carcinoma, rule out infections, reassure and give support'.[28] These principles for the management of mastalgia were followed almost exclusively for the subsequent 30 years. Audit of results has proved that reassurance alone was sufficient for 85% of cases, but medication has to be considered for the others.[38]

## Medical treatment

As cyclical premenstrual mastalgia was believed to be due to periodic salt and water retention[39-41] diuretics were widely prescribed for it.[42-44] In one of the few controlled trials in which an effect of diuretics for cyclical symptoms was shown, only women who had a premenstrual weight gain of at least 6.6 kg in two consecutive pretreatment cycles were selected.[45] Such patients are unusual amongst a cohort of women with mastalgia in whom isotope studies of total body water showed no consistent association between water retention and the symptoms.[46] Thus there is little scientific rationale for prescribing diuretics for cyclical mastalgia. Furthermore, two double blind placebo controlled studies showed no benefit from these.[47, 48] Diuretic therapy may even be counterproductive by inducing depression[49-51] or rebound oedema, or both, which may exacerbate the condition for which the treatment was originally given.[52]

Hormonal measures have been the most popular of the medical regimens for mastalgia.[53-58] This is almost certainly because a hormonal aetiology for the symptom is indicated by the fact that a substantial proportion of patients with mastalgia experienced this in a cyclical pattern. Various hormonal manipulations have been reported as being beneficial, including extracts of corpus luteum,[53, 59] testosterone[55, 60, 61,] and the radical step of oophorectomy.[62] The precise endocrine abnormality which these manoeuvres were intended to modify has been and still remains controversial. Some workers have postulated excessive stimulation of the breasts by over activity of the corpus luteum,[63, 64] while others have regarded the abnormality as relative hyperestrinism with reduced function of the corpus luteum.[1, 65, 66] Oestrogen supplementation was tried and fortunately fairly quickly abandoned.[34] Progestogens, initially as 'corpus luteum extract'[53, 59] have long had their advocates,[56, 66] but a recent placebo controlled trial of low dose medroxyprogesterone acetate did not show a significant improvement with this progestogen.[67]

Vitamin B_{6}, pyridoxine, which has benefited patients with the premenstrual syndrome, has also been tested for mastalgia relief; although there is a possible benefit for relief of mild tenderness this did not cause significant improvement in patients with severe symptoms in a randomised controlled trial.[90]

Most drug treatments for mastalgia which are currently in use or under evaluation are designed to affect the endocrine system, and may therefore be expected to be more useful for cyclical than for non-cyclical symptoms. These drugs are bromocriptine, danazol, γ-linolenic acid, goserelin, and tamoxifen.

## Bromocriptine

Bromocriptine is a dopamine agonist. It is absorbed when taken orally, stimulates release of dopamine from the posterior pituitary, and thereby inhibits release of prolactin. By this means it has a role in suppressing lactation and is useful in certain hyperprolactinaemic states such as galactorrhoea. In 1975 in open study it was reported to be effective in relieving breast pain.[57] This result was confirmed in cyclical mastalgia when bromocriptine was compared with placebo in a double blind trial.[68] In patients whose serum prolactin concentrations are ostensibly normal (as in the vast majority of women who experience cyclical mastalgia), bromocriptine tends to cause headaches and postural hypotension. To minimise these side effects treatment is started with a low dose (2.5 mg) at night and increased by gradual increments until the maintenance dose of 5 mg twice daily is achieved. A suitable regimen is: days 1 and 2 bromocriptine 2.5 mg at night, days 3 and 4 bromocriptine 2.5 mg twice daily, days 5 and 6 bromocriptine 2.5 mg in the morning and 5 mg at night, and day 7 onwards, bromocriptine 5 mg twice daily.

The length of time for which bromocriptine will be required cannot be predicted. An initial period of three months is a suitable time as long as the patient tolerates the tablets. No long term toxic effects of treatment with bromocriptine for cyclical mastalgia have been reported.

## Danazol

Danazol inhibits the secretion of the gonadotrophin luteinising hormone and follicle stimulating hormone (which in men is interstitial cell stimulating hormone). It acts to inhibit ovulation, development of the corpora lutea, and menstruation. Chemically, danazol can be thought of as an impeded androgen, and its principle indication is for treating endometriosis. It was shown in a pilot study in 1977, however, that it reduced breast discomfort.[58] Subsequently a double blind randomised crossover trial showed it to produce a significant reduction in cyclical mastalgia compared with placebo.[69, 70] It is as effective in this as bromocriptine.[71] As it suppresses menstruation, however, many clinicians use it for no more than three months at a time. Its potential side effects include nausea, flushing, weight gain, and the fact that it may be mildly androgenic. No serious toxicity after long term use for endometriosis has been reported. A suitable dose for treating cyclical mastalgia is 100 mg twice daily, although a smaller dose may be as effective; this has yet to be evaluated.[72].

*γ-linolenic acid*

This is a polyunsaturated essential fatty acid. It is a precursor of E series prostaglandins which have been postulated as effecting negative feedback in body reactions stimulated by prolactin.[73] This hypothesis assumes that cyclical mastalgia is an exaggerated response in breasts to stimulation by prolactin, the normal negative feedback of which is impaired by marginal deficiency of prostaglandin E1, itself resulting from dietary deficiency of γ-linolenic acid (Fig. 3.3). The initial clinical observation was made when women who were taking oil of the evening primrose (which is a rich natural source of γ-linolenic acid) for dietary reasons reported that their breasts were less tender premenstrually. A prospective placebo controlled trial comparing evening primrose oil with placebo showed a significant benefit from the oil containing γ-linolenic acid in those women whose mastalgia was cyclical, but not in those with non-cyclical symptoms.[74, 75]

*Goserelin*

Goserelin is an LH/RH analogue. Its action in the body is to increase secretion of both lutenising hormone and follicle stimulating hormone. If administered constantly it results in depletion of stores of both these hormones to such an extent that the menstrual cycle and ovulation cease. It acts when given continuously, therefore, as an antigonadotrophin such as danazol, but by a different mechanism. A formulation of goserelin has recently been devised in which a constant sustained release of the drug can be achieved from a depot injection in the subcutaneous fat.[76] As studies of the natural history of cyclical mastalgia show that this disappears after the menopause, and in view of the efficacy of the antigonadotrophin drug danazol in relieving cyclical mastalgia, theoretically the induction of an artificial (albeit temporary) menopause by goserelin might make this useful as a treatment for severe cyclical mastalgia. A randomised sham controlled evaluation of this is presently proceeding. From experience so far it seems

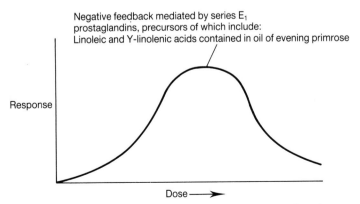

**Fig 3.3**   Dose response curve of prolactin mediated pathways.

that the induction of an artificial menopause is frequently accompanied by a pronounced reduction in cyclical mastalgia. The questions which remain to be answered by the full evaluation concern the length of remission of mastalgia and whether there are any serious short or long term side effects.

### Tamoxifen

Tamoxifen is an antioestrogen that works by blocking oestrogen receptors at target organs with a 'parodoxical' rise in peripheral oestradiol in premenopausal women. It has proven worth in the management of breast cancer but has also been shown to improve cyclical pain and nodularity significantly in a placebo controlled trial.[77] The mechanism of activity is uncertain but may be more related to associated falls in prolactin concentrations. Although further studies have failed to show important side effects, particularly on bone metabolism,[78] there are many who feel this drug should be reserved for malignant disease and only used otherwise in special circumstances.

## Surgical management

Operation has no part to play in the management of cyclical pronounced or cyclical prolonged mastalgia. 'Subcutaneous incisions throughout the gland as recommended by a French surgeon' were deprecated in Britain by Birkett in 1850.[79] Delbet advised mastectomy for painful breasts in which diffuse lumpiness was present.[80] Occasionally a patient with persistent pronounced mastalgia forces mastectomy to be considered. Where the pain is clearly cyclical, ablative surgery should be resisted if the indication is pain alone. If additional factors are present, particularly atypical epithelial hyperplasia[81] or even very strong family history of mammary malignancy, mastectomy might be contemplated but with recognition that the indication for mastectomy is not solely the attempt to relieve mastalgia but to prevent possible future malignancy. Mastectomy for cyclical mastalgia is rarely a solution to the complaints of the patient.[22]

There are several indications for surgical management of non-cyclical mastalgia, different indictions requiring different procedures. Having excluded a non-breast cause for non-cyclical mastalgia, the differential diagnosis for this symptom can be used as a diagnostic sieve (Table 3.2).

Duct ectasia which causes persistent and troublesome mastalgia can be treated by subareolar duct excision.[82-84] When this procedure is advised, patients should be informed that the sensation of the nipple on the operated side may be permanently altered. The operation results in reduction in mastalgia in a similar proportion of patients as are relieved of the other symptoms of duct ectasia for which the procedure is the accepted management. Fat necrosis, or a scar where trauma has occurred to a breast, can be treated by local excision of the site at which pain is experienced. For this to achieve its objective – that is remove the pain – two principles should be observed. Firstly, the incision should be made so that the resulting scar will be in or parallel to the Langer's lines of election.[85] In order to achieve this it

**Table 3.2** The clinical and radiological features that usually accompany the four most common benign patterns of non-cyclical mastalgia

| Pattern | Clinical features | Radiological features |
| --- | --- | --- |
| Duct ectasia | Precisely localised | Areas of coarse calcification |
| Fat necrosis | History of trauma | Architectural deformity |
| Sclerosing adenosis | Spontaneous onset | Clusters of small areas of calcification |
| Tietze's syndrome | Enlarged cartilage | No abnormality on mammogram or chest x-ray picture |

may be necessary to use a V-Y or a Z-plasty. Secondly, fastidious technique must be used to ensure that no haematoma follows the excision, for such a complication is itself a cause of non-cyclical mastalgia.[86]

Sclerosing adenosis as a cause of, or in strong association with, non-cyclical mastalgia may be suspected when the mammograms of a patient with this complaint show small areas of calcification (Fig. 3.1). These may be few and closely aggregated in a localised cluster, or many and widely scattered throughout the breast (Fig. 3.4). Such small areas of calcification are radiologically indistinguishable from those which are seen in 40 to 60% of mammograms of breasts containing carcinoma. It is mandatory, therefore, to biopsy the breast tissue containing these areas of calcification. Where a palpable mass is present at the tender locus this is done as a straight-

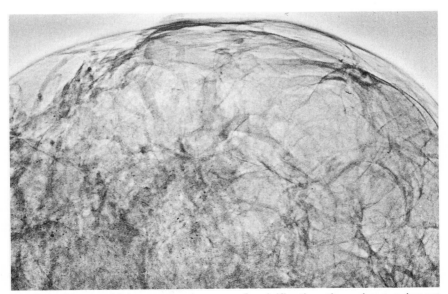

**Fig 3.4** Many widely scattered areas of calcification throughout a breast shown on a xero-mammogram of a patient with sclerosing adenosis.

forward breast biopsy, but with paraffin histology, because sclerosing adenosis is well known to mimic adenocarcinoma on frozen section.[87] When the area of calcification is not at the site of a palpable mass in the breast, a localising biposy is necessary to remove it for histological examination.[88, 89] The object is to confirm or refute malignant disease suspected from the mammogram. Where the histopathological diagnosis proves to be sclerosing adenosis, the pain with which the patient presented often disappears with removal of the calcified focus. This may be due to the reassurance th patient receives from the benign report, or from the removal of a pain inducing lesion. In order to minimise the likelihood of mastalgia developing later at the site of the localising biopsy, the two principles enunciated above should be strictly observed (namely that the incision should be in – or parallel to – a skin crease, and haemostasis should be meticulous).

## References

1. Geschickter CF. The endocrine aspects of chronic cystic mastitis. *Southern Surgeon* 1941; **10**: 457–86.
2. Saner FD. *The Breast*. Bristol: John Wright, 1950, p. 122.
3. Sutherland H, Stewart I. A critical analysis of the premenstrual syndrome. *Lancet* 1965; **i**: 1180–83.
4. Nichols S, Waters WE, Wheeler MJ. Management of female breast disease by Southampton general practitioners. *Br Med J* 1980; **281**: 1450–53.
5. Tietze A. Ueber eine eigenortige Höufung von fällen mit Dystrophie der Rippenknorpee *Berliner Klinische Wochenschrift* 1921; **58**: 829–31.
6. Ingelby H, Gershon–Cohen J. *Comparative Anatomy, Pathology and Roentgenology of the Breast*. Philadelphia, University of Pennsylvania Press, 1960, p. 247.
7. Evans KT, Gravelle IH. *Mammography, Thermography and Ultrasonography in Breast Disease*. London, Butterworth & Company Ltd, 1973, p. 75.
8. Foote FW, Stewart FW. Comparative studies of cancerous versus non-cancerous breasts. *Ann Surg* 1945; **121**: 6–53.
9. McDivitt RW, Stewart FW, Berg JW. Tumours of the breast. In: *Atlas of Tumour Pathology*. 2nd series, Fascicle 2, Washington, US Armed Forces, 1968, pp. 133–137.
10. Davies JD. Neural invasion in benign mammary dysplasia. *J Pathol* 1973; **109**: 225–31.
11. Taylor HB, Norris HJ. Epithelial invasion of nerves in benign disease of the breast. *Cancer* 1967; **20**: 2245–49.
12. Eusebi U, Azzopardi JC. Vascular infiltration in benign breast disease. *J Pathol* 1976; **118**: 9–16.
13. Preece PE, Fortt RW, Gravelle IH, *et al*. Some clinical aspects of sclerosing adenosis. *Clinical Oncology* 1979; **2**: 192.
14. Billroth CAT. *Handbook of Women's Diseases*. Vol. 2. Stuttgart, F. Enke, 1879, pp. 35–39.
15. Lane–Claypon JE. A further report on cancer of the breast with special reference to its associated antecedent conditions. *Report on Public Health and Medical Subjects* 1926; **32**: 1–189.
16. Cole WH, Rossiter LJ. Chronic cystic mastitis with particular reference to classification. *Ann Surg* 1944; **119**: 573–90.
17. Corry DC. Pain in carcinoma of the breast. *Lancet* 1952; **i**: 274–76.

18. Preece PE, Baum M, Mansel RE, *et al*. Importance of mastalgia in operable breast cancer. *Br Med J* 1982; **284**: 1299–1300.
19. Velpeau A. *A Treatise on the Diseases of the Breast and Mammary Region*. London, Sydenham Society, 1856, pp. 424–27.
20. River L, Silverstein J, Grout J, *et al*. Carcinoma of the breast: the diagnostic significance of pain. *Am J Surg* 1951; **82**: 733–35.
21. Atkins HJB. Pain in the breast. *Lancet* 1952; **i**: 271–74.
22. Hinton CP. Breast pain. In: Blamey RW. (Ed) *Complications in the Management of Breast Disease*. London, Bailliere Tindall, 1986, p. 236.
23. Farrow JH. Clinical considerations and treatment of in situ lobular breast cancer. *AJR* 1968; **120**: 652–56.
24. Bryant T. *The Diseases of the Breast*. London, Cassell and Co., 1887, p. 5.
25. Kumar S, Mansel RE, Hughes LE, *et al*. Prolactin response to thyrotropin releasing hormone stimulation and dopaminergic inhibition in benign breast disease. *Cancer* 1984; **53**: 1311–15.
26. Peters F, Schuth W, Schurech B, Breckwoldt M. Serum prolactin levels in patients with fibrocystic breast disease. *Obstet Gynecol* 1984; **64**: 381–85.
27. Kumar S, Mansel RE, Hughes LE, *et al*. Prediction of response to endocrine therapy in pronounced cyclical mastalgia using dynamic tests of prolactin release. *Clin Endocrinol* 1985; **23**: 699–704.
28. Geschickter CF. Mastodynia (painful breasts). In: *Diseases of the Breasts*. 2nd ed. Philadelphia, JB Lippincott Co., 1945, pp. 183–99.
29. Wisbey JR, Kumar S, Mansel RE, *et al*. Natural history of breast pain. *Lancet* 1983; **ii**: 672–74.
30. Hughes LE, Mansel E. Benign breast disease. In: Russell RCG. (Ed) *Recent Advances in Surgery 11*. Edinburgh, Churchill Livingstone, 1982, pp. 928–31.
31. Cooper A. *Illustrations of the Diseases of the Breast, Part 1*. London, Longman, Rees, Orme, Brown and Green, 1829, p. 76.
32. Velpeau A. *A Treatise on the Diseases of the Breast and Mammary Region*. London, Sydenham Society, 1856, p. 208.
33. Keynes G. Chronic mastitis. *Br J Surg* 1923; **11**: 89–121.
34. Atkins HJB. Chronic mastitis. *Lancet* 1938; **i**: 707–12.
35. Patey DH. Two common non-malignant conditions of the breast. *Br Med J* 1949; **i**: 96–99.
36. Haagensen CD. *Diseases of the Breast*, 2nd ed. Philadelphia, WB Saunders Co., 1971, p. 101.
37. Jeffcoate N. *Principles of Gynaecology*. 4th ed. London, Butterworths, 1975, p. 550.
38. Pye JK, Mansel RE, Hughes LE. Clinical experience of drug treatments for mastalgia. *Lancet* 1985; **ii**: 373–77.
39. Taylor HC. The relation of chronic mastitis to certain hormones of the ovary and pituitary and to co-incident gynaecological lesions. Part 1: Theoretical considerations and histological studies. *Surg Gynecol Obstet* 1936; **62**: 129–48.
40. Geiringer E. Mittelwahn. A reconsideration of pre-menstrual phenomena. *Journal of Obstetrics and Gynaecology of the British Empire* 1951; **58**: 1010–18.
41. Swan R. The pre-menstrual syndrome. *Lancet* 1965; **ii**: 41.
42. Israel SL. *Menstrual Disorders and Sterility*. 5th ed. New York, Harper and Row, 1967, p. 171.
43. Winterton WR. Painful breasts during menstruation. *Practitioner* 1969; **202**: 178.
44. Idiopathic oedema of women. *Br Med J* 1976; **i**: 979–80.
45. Werch A, Kane RE. Treatment of pre-menstrual tension with metolazone: a

double blind evaluation of a new diuretic. *Current Therapeutic Research 1976;* **19:** 565–71.

46. Preece PE, Richards AR, Owen GM, Hughes LE. Mastalgia and total body water. *Br Med J* 1975; **4:** 498–500.
47. Jordheim O. The pre-menstrual syndrome. *Acta Obstet Gynecol Scand* 1972; **51:** 77–80.
48. Modell W. *Drugs of Choice.* 1974–75 ed. St. Louis, CV Mosby Co., 1974, p. 79.
49. Hullin RP, Bailley AD, McDonald R, *et al.* Variations in body water during recovery from depression. *Br J Psychiatry* 1967; **113:** 573–83.
50. Hullin RP, Bailley AD, McDonald R, *et al.* Body water variations in manic depressive psychosis. *Br J Psychiatry* 1967; **113:** 584–92.
51. Herzberg BN. Body composition and pre-menstrual tension. *J Psychosom Res* 1971; **15:** 251–57.
52. MacGregor GA, Markandu ND, Roulston JE, *et al.* Is 'idiopathic' oedema idiopathic? *Lancet* 1979; **i:** 3397–400.
53. Lisser H. A note on the use of corpus luteum to prevent the painful breasts of menstruation. *Endocrinology* 1918; **2:** 12–15.
54. Spence AW. Testosterone proprionate in chronic mastitis. *Lancet* 1939; **ii:** 820–23.
55. Atkins HJB. Treatment of chronic mastitis. *Lancet* 1940; **ii:** 411–13.
56. Cunningham K, Lang WR. Result of a blind clinical trial conducted on 50 cases of hormonal mastopathy. *Med J Aust* 1962; **49:** 341–44.
57. Shulz KD, del Pozo E, Lose KH, *et al.* Successful treatment of mastodynia with the prolactin inhibitor bromocriptine (CB154). *Archiv fur Gynakologie* 1975; **220:** 83–87.
58. Ash RH, Greenblatt RB. The use of an impeded androgen danazol in the treatment of benign breast disorders. *Am J Obstet Gynecol* 1977; **127:** 130–34.
59. Samuel M. Mastodynia. *Zentralbl Gynakol* 1928; **52:** 1267–68.
60. Tailhefer A. Résultats du traitement de quelques mastopathies par le proprionate de testostérone. *Paris Medical* 1938; **2:** 189–91.
61. Desmarest D. Le traitement des mastopathies par la testostérone. *La Semaine des Hopitaux de Paris* 1938; **14:** 251–63.
62. Leriche M. Hypertrophie mammaire douloureuse, flétrie par castration. *Lyon Chirurgie* 1923; **20:** 653–655.
63. Cutler M. The cause of painful breasts and treatment by means of ovarian residue. *JAMA* 1931; **96:** 1201–205.
64. Bertner EW. Painful breasts: a gynecological problem. *Texas State Journal of Medicine* 1932; **28:** 528–31.
65. Pollosson E, Mathieu J, Haour P. Etude de la cytologie vaginale dans les seins douloureux. *Gynaecologie et Obstetrique* 1951; **50:** 260–64.
66. Sitrak–Ware LR, Sterkers N, Mowszowicz I, Mauvais-Jarvis P. Inadequate corpus luteal function in women with benign breast disease. *J Clin Endocrinol Metab* 1977; **44:** 7771–74.
67. Maddox P, Mansel RE, Horobin JM, *et al.* Low dose medroxyprogesterone acetate for mastalgia. *Br J Surg.* 1989; **76.**
68. Mansel RE, Preece PE, Hughes LE. A double blind trial of the prolactin inhibitor bromocriptine in painful benign breast disease. *Br J Surg* 1978; **65:** 724–27.
69. Mansel RE, Wisbey JR, Hughes LE. The use of danazol in the treatment of painful benign breast disease – preliminary results. *Postgrad Med J* 1979; **55** (Suppl. 5): 61–65.
70. Mansel RE, Wisbey JR, Hughes LE. Controlled trial of the antigonadotrophin danazol in painful and nodular benign breast disease. *Lancet* 1982; **i:** 928–30.

71. Hinton CP, Bishop HM, Holliday HW, *et al*. A double-blind controlled trial of danazol and bromocriptine in the management of severe cyclical breast pain. *Br J Clin Pract* 1986; **40**: 326–30.
72. Harrison BJ, Maddox PR, Mansel RE. Maintenance therapy of cyclical mastalgia using low dose danazol. *J R Coll Surg Edinb* 1989; **34**: 79–81.
73. Horrobin DF. Cellular basis of prolactin action: relevance to breast cancer and the menstrual cycle. *Med Hypotheses* 1979; **5**: 599–620.
74. Preece PE, Hanslip JI, Gilbert L, *et al*. Evening primrose oil (Efamol) for mastalgia. In: Horrobin DF. (Ed) *Clinical Uses of Essential Fatty Acid*. Montreal, Eden, 1982, pp. 147–154.
75. Preece PE. Endocrine therapy of benign breast disease. In: Timothy A. (Ed) *Place of Endocrine Therapy in Breast Disease*. London, Royal Society of Medicine, 1987, pp. 78–79.
76. Hutchinson FG, Furr BJA. Biodegradable polymers for the sustained release of peptides. *Biochem Soc Trans* 1985; **13**: 520–23.
77. Fentima. IS, Caleffi M, Brame K, *et al*. Double blind controlled trial of tamoxifen therapy for mastalgia. *Lancet* 1986; **i**: 287–88.
78. Fentiman IS, Caleffi M, Murby B, Fogelman I. Dosage, duration and short term effect on bone mineral content of tamoxifen treatment of mastalgia. *Br J Clin Pract* 1988; **42** (Suppl. 56): 18–20.
79. Birkett J. *The Diseases of the Breast and their Treatment*. London, Longman, Brown, Green and Longmans, 1850, p. 164.
80. Delbet P. Mamelle: troubles nerveux–mastodynie. In: Duplay S, Reclus P. (Eds) *Traité de Chirurgie*, Vol. V. 2nd ed. Paris, Masson et Cie, 1898, pp. 865–69.
81. Page DL, Dupont WE, Rogers LW, Rados MS. Atypical hyperplastic lesions of the female breast: a long term follow-up study. *Cancer 1985*; **55**: 2698–708.
82. Hadfield GJ. Excision of the major duct system for benign disease of the breast. *Br J Surg* 1960; **47**: 472–77.
83. Urban JA. Excision of the major duct system of the breast. *Cancer* 1963; **16**: 516–520.
84. Hadfield GJ. Further experience of the operation for excision of the major duct system of the breast. *Br J Surg* 1968; **55**: 531–35.
85. Langer C. *Lehrbuch der Anatomie des Menschen. (Textbook of Human Anatomy)*. Vienna, W Braumuller, 1865.
86. Preece PE, Hughes LE, Mansel RE, *et al*. Clinical syndromes of mastalgia. *Lancet* 1976; **ii**: 670–73.
87. Urban JA, Adair FE. Sclerosing adenosis. *Cancer* 1949; **2**: 625–34.
88. Frank HA, Hall FM, Steer ML. Preoperative localisation of non-palpable breast lesions demonstrated by mammography. *N Engl J Med* 1976; **295**: 259–60.
89. Preece PE. Localising technique for impalpable breast lesions. In: Walker WF. (Ed) *A Colour Atlas of Minor Surgery*. London, Wolfe Medical Publications Ltd, 1986, 97–99.
90. Smallwood J, Ah-Kye D, Taylor I. Vitamin $B_6$ in the treatment of premenstrual mastalgia. *Br J Clin Pract* 1986; **40**: 532–34.

# 4

# Fibroadenosis

P McCULLOCH AND WD GEORGE

## The problem

Fibroadenosis is a term that refers to a clinical syndrome rather than a specific histological abnormality; it has survived in clinical usage mainly through convenience, but also because a more accurate alternative based on scientific data has never been found.

The syndrome can be defined as a 'diffuse benign condition of the premenopausal breast characterised by lumpiness and irregularity of breast tissue, with or without pain, that predominates in the latter half of the menstrual cycle'. More simply this represents 'painful nodularity'.

## Epidemiology

Some degree of clinically detectable lumpiness is such a frequent finding in premenopausal women that it cannot be considered abnormal.[1] Factors which cause such changes to be brought to medical attention are many and varied; the degree of lumpiness and its fluctuation with the menstrual cycle vary greatly among women, and those with more pronounced changes and those with more persistent lumpiness are more likely to present to their doctor. In the same way those in whom lumpiness occurs only in one area or is asymmetrical are more likely to become concerned than the majority in whom the condition is bilateral and symmetrical. Often the association of the lumpiness with pain, either premenstrually or at unpredictable times through the cycle, is the deciding factor in causing the patient to become concerned.

As well as these objective factors, attitudes to (and education about) health and health care play an important part in deciding which women ignore the changes in their breasts and which become concerned about them. There is little or no factual information about class differences in the incidence of fibroadenosis.

In view of this multiplicity of influences that determine which women seek medical advice, it is not surprising that estimates of the incidence of fibroadenosis vary widely. It is more important to note, however, that these estimates range between 30 and 100% of women in the 20–45 age group. This confirms that the mere presence of lumpiness in the breasts is not abnormal in a statistical or pathological sense. Indeed, where pain is taken as the major symptom, one study from Liverpool has shown an incidence of significant breast pain in two thirds of a screened population.[2]

## Pathophysiology

It is traditionally believed that fibroadenosis is caused either by an imbalance in the hormones which normally control breast tissue or by an abnormal response of the target tissue to normal hormonal influences.[3] The control of mammary epithelial growth by the interaction of oestrogen, progesterone, and prolactin (together with other hormones) is far from understood; oestrogenic influences cause the proliferation of duct epithelium with lengthening and branching of ducts and an increase in their calibre. Progesterone inhibits this oestrogenic effect while promoting differentiation of the breast acini. Prolactin, in association with other hormones, promotes lactation, but also has important influences on the pattern of proliferation of the breast epithelium, partly because its capacity for inducing luteal insufficiency decreases progesterone secretion. Women who have anovulatory cycles, whether at the extremes of menstrual activity or as a result of treatment with danazol, are less likely to suffer from fibroadenosis.

Consistent differences in the hormonal patterns of menstruating women with and without fibroadenosis have proved subtle and difficult to identify; hormone assay techniques have not always been sensitive and the pulsatile nature of steroid hormone release has made measurements related to time difficult.

Early studies suffered greatly from lack of definition of the study group and poor patient selection. The results of Sitrak–Ware *et al*,[4] which claimed to show a relative progesterone deficiency, highlighted a further problem – that of random assays at non-synchronised times in the menstrual cycle. Careful studies with daily sampling[5] have since failed to support these earlier findings and the so called 'luteal deficiency' theory has fallen from favour.

Dynamic studies of prolactin secretion[6] have provided the strongest clue so far; the Cardiff group (and others since) have shown that the peak secretion of prolactin in response to thyrotrophin releasing hormone is higher in defined groups of patients with either cyclical mastalgia or nodularity alone than in well matched controls; the basal concentrations in both groups remained normal. How this subtle endocrine abnormality translates into symptoms and signs within the breast is still unknown. An ultrasound assessment of breast structure according to peaks of thyrotrophin releasing hormone secretion has failed to show any structural difference, but this may not be the ideal probe.[7]

Several groups have looked at the effects of caffeine[8] and the methyl xanthines but these do not appear to relate significantly to fibroadenosis, although adrenalin concentrations have been shown to be raised in mastalgia patients. Further data, particularly on 'cause and effect' are required here before further conclusions can be drawn.

The mechanism of any 'endocrine fault' may be suggested by the pharmacology of the agents that have been proved to alter the natural history of this complaint. Danazol, bromocriptine, evening primrose oil, tamoxifen and a low fat diet undoubtedly help symptoms, but their specific mechanism of action is largely unknown because many different relevant steroid groups are affected. In a recent review Goodwin *et al*[9] attempted to correlate these effects, and hypothesised that there is an underlying fault of lipid metabolism within the breast, mediated by prolactin secretion.

The possibility that faults in the target tissue may be responsible has long been considered, but ethical considerations have severely limited study to routine histological examination from biopsy or post mortem study.

## Histopathology

Standard surgical texts list many histological abnormalities associated with fibroadenosis; these invariably include fibrosis, adenosis, cyst formation, and epithelial hyperplasia. There is, however, little scientific evidence that these histological features are truly 'pathological' or that they correlate with symptoms and signs (see chapter 1). Love *et al* in 1982 recognised this and were moved to say that fibrocystic disease, (or fibroadenosis), is a 'non-disease'.[10] What has tended to happen over the years is that earnest attempts by pathologists have been made to correlate histological appearances with the clinical features. Each has laid emphasis on their own interpretation of features, with little regard to what other 'asymptomatic' areas of the breast may be like. Surgeons have been less than critical in accepting these correlations, perhaps because they justify or confirm the need to biopsy in the first place.

There are no consistent and scientifically proved histological abnormalities that account for the nodularity and pain associated with this condition. Oedema or fluid retention has been suggested, but this is not supported by studies on fluid balance, and the failure of diuretics to improve symptoms makes it most unlikely. It seems likely that a subtle change in stromal ground substance not identified by gross study of body fluids may account for both nodularity and pain.

## Cancer risk

It has become entrenched within the minds of clinicians that fibroadenosis indicates a higher than normal risk of developing breast cancer probably through misleading and confused reports on the subject. This is highlighted in a historical review by Azzopardi,[11] who clearly shows this to be due to intractable problems of classification and definition.

The evidence falls into four categories. First, there is the common association of both fibroadenosis and cancer with parity. In premonopausal women both are somewhat commoner in those who are nulliparous, but this of course does not necessarily imply that the one predisposes to the other. Secondly, there is the undeniable similarity between early forms of preinvasive carcinoma and the more florid changes of epithelial proliferation which may incidentally be seen in breast biopsy material. Some authors see this as evidence of a gradual progression of abnormalities beginning with hyperplasia and graduating through dysplasia to neoplasia, as has been described in other epithelial tissues. The third point, that of the physical association of breast cancer with fibroadenotic tissue (whatever this may be) is one on which the available evidence is scanty: the evidence that exists does not support the theory that cancer arises much more frequently in abnormal breast tissue. The final point, that of a positive association between the presence of fibroadenosis and the development of cancer, is one on which much work has been done. Most papers on the subject do describe an increased risk of cancer in these patients. The work of Dupont and Page[12] has been invaluable in elucidating this problem. They have successfully defined a subgroup of patients who are at an increased risk of subsequent cancer. This subgroup is, however, small and the remaining considerable majority of patients are at no excess risk compared with the normal population. The distinct and well defined changes of atypical lobular hyperplasia and atypical ductal hyperplasia are associated with a cancer risk of up to 11 times that of the normal population. Fibroadenosis *per se*, without these specific histological findings, poses no increased risk.

## Diagnosis

The diagnosis of fibroadenosis can usually be made on clinical grounds but an element essential to the successful management of patients is the positive reassurance that there is no malignancy; to this end many clinicians reasonably use further investigations such as mammography and cytology.

A history of tenderness associated with 'congestion' or lumpiness that is worse in the second half of the cycle is typical. Most will feel this in the outer half of the breast and often into the axilla or arm. Symptoms are often bilateral, with one side worse than the other.

Patients are commonly between 20 and 40 years old, but a further group present in the perimenopausal phase probably as a result of true hormonal imbalance. A history of mild premenstrual tenderness is not always obtained and attacks frequently occur out of the blue; in some, a stressful time such as a home move or bereavement can closely synchronise with the onset, which lends support to a hypothalamic pituitary aetiology. There is little evidence that affected patients exhibit personality disorders or neuroses as suggested in historical texts. Preece has shown these patients to be no different from non-sufferers.[13]

Patients should preferably be examined during the first half of the menstrual cycle and on two separate occasions; changes in areas of nodularity and tenderness between two times strongly support a diagnosis of fibroadenosis. Other important features are the bilateral changes and their predominance in the upper outer quadrant.

Making the distinction between a true lump or discrete mass and areas of thickening or nodularity is usually straightforward but needs experience. Before making decisions on management which could lead to unnecessary biopsy and psychological morbidity, patients should be reviewed by an experienced clinician.

## Investigation

Investigations which help diagnose fibroadenosis do so essentially by excluding other serious disease, because as already stated this is a clinical syndrome. The exclusion of cancer in this way is clearly of benefit in the 'active reassurance' element of treatment. Investigations currently used by clinicians include fine needle aspiration cytology, mammography, and ultrasonography.

### Fine needle aspiration cytology

Needle aspiration and subsequent cytology of plaques of 'fibroadenosis' are generally unrewarding; it is difficult to obtain a cellular smear mainly because the underlying tissue has no focus of densely cellular material, and is histologically normal. Where clinical doubt exists, several smears that show no malignant cells – when considered with other negative results – may help to prevent unnecessary biopsy.

### Mammography

This is probably the single most important investigation, for its 'normality' in the patient's eyes provides the greatest reassurance; paradoxically the premenopausal breast may show such marked stromal density that any evidence of carcinoma could be lost within it. Nevertheless, in patients over 30 years old, in whom the use of X-rays on the breast is generally acceptable, the finding of a normal mammogram (particularly in high risk patients such as those with a positive family history) can be very reassuring to the clinician. In those under 30 in whom the risk of cancer is small, breast ultrasonography is an effective alternative to mammography; it does not pick up small areas of calcification, so in those rare cases of high cancer risk mammography may still be justified.

### Breast ultrasonography

This is mentioned briefly, as a full and critical account of its use in the breast in given in chapter 2. It is a safe technique which has the advantage of repeated use without risk. In premenopausal breasts, particularly in the younger age group, ultrasonography can see through X-ray density and resolve focal abnormalities which may otherwise be invisible. It is highly sensitive for cysts, good for fibroadenomas, and has a greater sensitivity for clinically suspected carcinomas than mammography.[14] Like all radiological techniques it has limitations, with varying rates of false positive and false negative diagnoses (see chapter 2).

## Treatment

Fibroadenosis is a condition that should be managed conservatively; patients must be actively reassured that there is no serious disease or cancer risk. Lumpiness or nodularity for it own sake requires no specific treatment; patients should be properly counselled and reviewed 2 or 3 months later during the first half of a cycle. If all is well they can be discharged. It is of immense value that patients within this category be seen finally by a consultant or senior member of the team who can make this decision with judgement and authority. If pain is the most serious symptom then treatment should still be on conservative lines, although a few may benefit from specific drugs; such patients are dealt with in detail in the preceding chapter on mastalgia. Open biopsy should be avoided unless there are good grounds, as scar tissue itself causes pain and distortion and makes future assessment exceedingly difficult.

There are two groups of patients who merit special attention. Those in the perimenopausal group with other symptoms of hormone inbalance are in an age group in which the incidence of cancer is significantly higher. If after full investigation to exclude malignancy reasonable doubt still exists within a local area, then biopsy is mandatory; in other cases it may be prudent to follow up patients for longer both clinically and with further mammograms.

The second group are in a similar but older age group in which the cessation of ovarian activity has precipitated the need for oestrogen replacement. A small number of patients on 'combination' replacement treatment do suffer fibroadenosis-like symptoms and are referred for specialist advice. Their management is the same as in the perimenopausal group, with the added simple advice that they try the lowest dose preparation or stop it altogether. Many of the postmenopausal symptoms can be managed in other ways.

## Sclerosing adenosis

This condition is mentioned here because it is occasionally included in the fibroadenosis range of conditions, when it should not be. It has an undoubted histological identity which in some cases may be difficult for the pathologist to distinguish from malignancy, although it is entirely benign and without cancer risk. It is regarded by some[1] to be an aberration of normality rather than a disease, as the appearances would fit for breast tissue in which the process of cyclical change and involution in the stroma and epithelium has become disorganised.

Clinical interest lies in the extraordinary capacity of this lesion to mimic malignancy, not only histologically. Areas of sclerosing adenosis are invariably asymptomatic and picked up coincidentally in biopsy specimens, but are a recognised cause of localised non-cyclical discomfort. They can produce thickening or lumps, and even tether the skin if the sclerosing element pulls on surrounding breast structures. On mammography they can mimic cancers with ease and are a recognised pitfall; lesions such as these must always be biopsied, and making a purely clinical diagnosis of sclerosis adenosis must be avoided.

# Conclusion

'Fibroadenosis' is a poor term to use for a clinical condition without histological identity. It is nevertheless accepted in clinical usage and serves only in explanation to women who have pain and lumpiness as real symptoms. Management depends on the exclusion of cancer and cancer risk in a sympathetic setting with minimal use of biopsy. For those with persistent pain (mastalgia) drug treatment may occasionally be needed.

# References

1. Hughes LE, Mansel RE, Webster DJT. ANDI – a new perspective on benign breast disorders. *Br J Clin Pract* 1988; **42** (Suppl. 56): 1–9.
2. Leinster SJ, Whitehouse GH, Walsh PV. Cyclical mastalgia: clinical and mammograpic observations in a screened population. *Br J Surg* 1987; **74**: 220–22.
3. Mansel RE. Update on the treatment of fibroadenosis. *Br J Clin Pract* 1988; **42** (Suppl. 56): 12–17.
4. Sitrak–Ware L, Strekers N, Moszowicz I, Mauvais–Jarvis P. Inadequate corpus luteal function in women with benign breast disease. *J Clin Endocrinol Metab* 1977; **44**: 771–74.
5. Walsh PV, Bulbrook RO, Stell PM, *et al*. Serum progesterone concentration during the luteal phase in women with benign breast disease. *Eur J Cancer Clin Oncol* 1984; **20**: 1339–43.
6. Kumar S, Mansel RE, Hughes LE, *et al*. Prediction of response to endocrine therapy in pronounced cyclical mastaglia using dynamic tests of prolactin release. *Clin Endocrinol* 1985; **23**: 699–704.
7. Ayers WJT, Gidwani GP. The 'luteal breast' – hormonal and sonographic investigation of benign breast disease in patients with cyclical mastalgia. *Fertil Steril* 1983; **40**: 779–84.
8. Minton JP, Freeking MK, Webster DJT, Mathews RH. Caffeine, cyclic nucleotides and breast disease. *Surgery* 1979; **86**: 105–8.
9. Goodwin PJ, Neelam M, Boyd F. Cyclical mastopathy – a critical review of therapy. *Br J Surg* 1988; **75**: 837–44.
10. Love SM, Goleman RS, Silen W. Fibrocystic 'disease' of the breast – a non-disease. *N Engl J Med* 1982; **307**: 1010–14.
11. Azzopardi JG. Problems in breast pathology. London, WB Saunders, 1979: 92–105.
12. Dupont WD and Page DL. Risk factors for breast cancer in women with proliferative breast disease. *N Engl J Med* 1985; **312**: 146–51.
13. Preece PE, Mansel RE and Hughes LE. Mastalgia: psychoneurosis or organic disease? *Br Med J* 1978; **i**: 29–30.
14. Smallwood JA, Menegatti S, Guyer P, *et al*. The accuracy of ultrasound in diagnosis of breast masses. *Ann R Coll Surg Eng* 1986; **68**: 19–22.

# 5

# Cystic disease of the breast

JM DIXON

## Definition

Cystic disease of the breast is a term which has been used to describe a variety of conditions in which palpable breast cysts are the dominant feature. Palpable breast cysts may be accompanied by a host of microscopic lesions, including microcysts, apocrine change, adenosis, fibrosis, and epithelial hyperplasia. These microscopic changes have been previously considered pathological and have been given a variety of names including fibrocystic disease, fibroadenosis, chronic cystic mastitis, cystic epithelial hyperplasia, cystic mastopathy, benign mammary dysplasia, and Schimmelbusch's disease.[1, 2] It is now appreciated that microcysts, apocrine change, adenosis, fibrosis, and minimal and moderate degrees of hyperplasia are common findings in the period of breast involution,[3-6] and may be considered as a normal part of the involutional process. In the past, a patient with a localised clinical abnormality was often subjected to biopsy, and the histological changes listed above correlated with that clinical episode. This ignores both the frequency with which these features are present in patients without symptoms and the poor correlation between symptoms and histology.[4-6] These histological terms can therefore have no place in clinical practice and the term cystic disease should be restricted to the clearly defined group of women with clinically palpable breast cysts.

## History, origin and mode of formation

Astley Cooper in 1829 first distinguished cysts from malignancy.[7] The first comprehensive clinical and pathological descriptions of cystic disease were made over half a century later by Reclus[8] and Brissaud.[9] Reclus showed that his 'maladie kystique des mammelles' was frequently bilateral, might involve the whole of the gland, and that most cysts were impalpable. He regarded cysts as independent new formations.[8] In contrast, Brissaud[9] thought cysts arose by proliferation of lobular epithelium to form compact cellular masses which became cystic following central necrosis. This theory was later supported by Schimmelbusch.[10] König[11] considered cysts to be inflammatory in origin and called the condition chronic cystic mastitis, a term which is still unfortunately used by some clinicians today.

During the early part of the twentieth century it was believed that cysts arose as a consequence of senile involution of breast lobules.[12-14] An extreme proponent of the involutional theory was McFarland,[14] who considered cysts as variations of the involutional process of lactating lobules. Other workers[15] could find no evidence of residual lactational lobules and returned to the theory originally proposed by Reclus, that cysts were new formations arising from hyperplasia.

The role of apocrine epithelium in cystic disease was first recognised by Creighton.[16] The observation that cysts were frequently lined with this epithelium led to the view that cysts were derived from apocrine sweat glands. These glands were thought by some to be normally present in the breast[17, 18] and by others to be present as a result of a developmental anomaly.[19-20] Studies have now shown that apocrine epithelium is not present within the breast in early life.[21, 22] When present in later life, it can occur in direct continuity with normal ductal epithelium, making the theory that cysts originate in sweat glands untenable. It is now accepted that apocrine epithelium in the breast arises as a result of a transformation from normal lobular or ductal epithelium.[1] This transformation may or may not be a true metaplasia.[3, 22, 23] Although most cysts are lined with apocrine epithelium,[3] some are lined with flattened epithelium.[23-26]

It has been suggested that flattened cysts arise by simple lobular dilatation, whereas apocrine cysts arise from lobules in which apocrine change is already present.[24, 25] The composition of cyst fluids and lobular secretions, however, is not compatible with such an explanation.[27-29] Others believe all cysts arise from microcysts,[30] which have been reported to be exclusively apocrine.[25, 29-31] The mechanism by which two populations of macrocysts develop from a single population of microcysts is unknown.

In conclusion, palpable breast cysts appear to arise from lobules. Two major types exist, lined either by apocrine or flattened epithelium. Cysts develop during the period of breast involution and are best regarded as aberrations of the involutional process.[32] Their mode of formation and nature of their precursors remain uncertain.

## Natural history

### Incidence

Approximately 7% of all women in the western world present to hospital with a clinically palpable breast cyst.[3] The exact incidence is difficult to ascertain as results from post mortem studies of the breast fail to distinguish between microscopic and grossly visible cysts.[33] In a post mortem study of 225 patients, Frantz[4] reported 18.6% of patients had cysts 1 mm or more in diameter. Most of these were small and probably only one cyst (measuring 2 cm in diameter) was large enough to be palpable. In 34% of patients the microscopic lesions, microcysts, apocrine metaplasia, and epithelial proliferation were seen.

## Age incidence

The age distribution of patients with cysts is shown in Fig. 5.1. Cysts are most common in the 40–50 age group. Only 2.2% of patients with cysts are below the age of 30, and 1.8% are over 54 years of age. Cysts occur most frequently during the period of breast involution and least frequently in the period after the menopause.

## Number of cysts

The total number of cysts in individuals varies greatly (Table 5.1). Approximately half of all patients develop a single cyst, a third have from 2 to 5 cysts and the remainder develop more than 5.

## Breast affected

Cystic disease appears to be more common in the left breast than the right. In

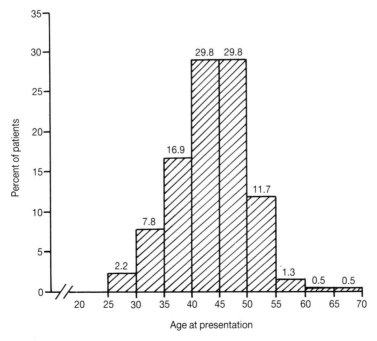

**Fig 5.1** Age distribution of patients presenting with breast cysts (from Haagensen et al[3]).

**Table 5.1** Total number of cysts in 1998 patients with cystic disease followed up for a minimum of five years (from Haagensen *et al*[3]).

| Number of cysts | % | |
|---|---|---|
| 1 | 48.8 | |
| 2 | 15.8 | |
| 3 | 9.1 | 33.5 |
| 4 | 5.4 | |
| 5 | 3.2 | |
| 6–25 | 15.8 | 17.9 |
| 26+ | 2.1 | |

a series of 2129 patients reported by Haagensen *et al*,[3] 36.7% of patients had cysts affecting only the left breast, 27.9% had cysts affecting only the right breast, and 35.4% had cysts in both breasts. It is of interest that breast carcinoma has also been reported to be more common in the left breast.[3]

## Aetiology of cystic disease

Hormones are the major factors in the development and growth of the normal breast and it follows that abnormalities in the gland may be a reflection of abnormalities in hormone concentrations. The evidence that cystic disease is hormonally related includes its bilateral nature, its relation to the menopause, and the response of cystic disease to endocrine treatment.[33-35]

There is no animal model for cystic disease so the only studies performed have been in humans. The problem with these studies is that the action of hormones on the breast is complex and it is likely that the action of any hormone is not directly related to the plasma concentration. It is more likely that there is an interaction between different hormones, the relative concentrations or balance being more important than absolute concentrations. It is perhaps then not surprising that studies which have measured individual hormones in patients with cystic disease have failed to find consistent abnormalities in plasma hormone concentrations. One study of patients with so called fibrocystic disease reported high concentrations of prolactin in patients after acute stimulation,[36] and others have shown there is an increased incidence of luteal phase insufficiency in these women,[37] the action of oestrogen in the luteal phase then being unopposed. The problems with these studies are a lack of definition of the patients studied and an inability of other centres to obtain similar results. Patients with cystic disease do not display consitent abnormalities in the plasma concentration of hormones.

Because measurement of hormones excreted in urine or circulating in the blood may not be a reflection of the endocrine environment within the breast itself, hormones have been measured in breast fluids. These studies have shown very high concentrations of hormones in some cysts.[28, 29]

Concentrations of hormones in breast secretions have also been reported to be many times higher than those seen in plasma, but no differences have been shown in the concentrations of hormones in the secretions of patients with different breast conditions.[27, 38]

## Clinical aspects of cystic disease

### Presentation

Patients with cystic disease usually present with smooth, discrete, breast lumps which may be fluctuant. The non-fluctuant so called 'tension' cysts may clinically resemble a breast carcinoma. Patients with cysts also present with breast pain, or the cysts may be discovered incidentally on clinical or mammographic examination, as part of the screening process.

If a breast lump is suspected to be a cyst, a needle aspirate (with a 21 g needle) should be carried out to confirm or refute the diagnosis; if a cyst is confirmed, then it should be aspirated completely. The aspirate from cysts varies in colour from pale yellow to dark green to brown; what causes the colour is not known.

Occasionally the fluid is bloodstained and only these specimens should be submitted for cytology, as it is now accepted that routine cytological examination of cyst fluid is unnecessary and potentially misleading.[39, 40] Carcinomas presenting as cysts are rare.[2, 41] They should be clearly separated from carcinomas adjacent to cysts which may be more common.[39] Cytology is only likely to be of value in intracystic carcinomas. The fluid from these is usually bloodstained.[39-41] An evenly bloodstained cyst aspirate is therefore a definite indication for excision biopsy. A carcinoma adjacent to a cyst may become palpable after aspiration and resolution of the cyst; this is suggested by a residual mass after cyst aspiration, although most residual masses will not be carcinomas. They may be nodular plaques of breast tissue containing microcysts, or they may be normal breast tissue which becomes palpable as a result of compression by the cyst. Any residual mass after cyst aspiration should be further investigated, either by aspiration cytology or by a further clinical examination 3 weeks later. If on review the mass is still present, or abnormal cells are obtained on cytology, it should be biopsied. Most patients with residual masses who do not have malignancy will be saved an unnecessary biopsy if this policy is adopted.

Patients with cystic disease who are over the age of 35 should have mammography, preferably performed immediately prior to the clinic visit. Cysts have characteristic mammographic appearances (Fig. 5.2), although they can be misinterpreted as malignant or suspicious lesions. The advantage of having mammograms available when the patient is first seen is that they may alert the clinician to the presence of either more cysts or some other lesion. The patient may then be saved false reassurance. More cysts are frequently present in the breasts and visible on X-ray than are clinically palpable. Cysts have been reported to occur more commonly in

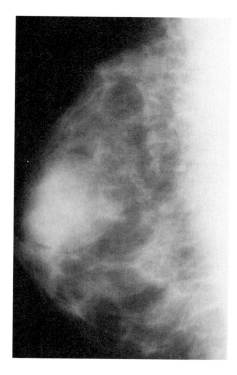

**Fig 5.2** Mammogram of a patient with a breast cyst. The halo around a clearly defined opacity are the characteristic mammographic features of a cyst.

mammographically dense (so called dysplastic) breasts. Where a lesion is seen on X-ray which is considered to be a cyst and it is impalpable, then ultrasound should be performed to confirm its cystic nature.

All patients should be reviewed 3 weeks after initial cyst aspiration and re-examined. Refilling of a cyst is not an indication for biopsy,[42] but a cyst which persistently refills rapidly on more than two occasions after aspiration should be excised as patients with cysts associated with breast cancer have been reported to refill their cysts.[39, 40] As previously indicated, most if not all patients with an intracystic carcinoma have either a bloodstained initial aspirate, a residual mass after aspiration, or both.[9, 40] The possibility that new cyst formation at the same site as the initial cyst aspiration may be more common than actual refilling of a cyst[29] is another argument against the view that cyst recurrence is an indication for biopsy.[39, 40] In previous series of patients with cysts associated with breast cancer, a number of patients were postmenopausal by more than five years. As previously noted, cysts in these women are uncommon so any patient presenting with a cyst more than 5 years after the menopause should be treated with particular care, and where there is clinical or mammographic suspicion, excisional biopsy should be performed.

Patients with recurrent or further cysts should have them re-aspirated at review, and the patient seen again at regular intervals until cysts are no longer palpable. Where no further cysts are palpable the patient can be discharged. As previously noted, 2% of all women with cysts develop large numbers of cysts. In these patients it may be unnecessary to aspirate every cyst which develops, providing that they are confirmed as cystic by ultrasound and the patient has all cysts aspirated at least once a year followed by a full clinical and mammographic examination.

## Treatment of multiple cysts

Multiple cyst formation can be arrested by treatment with danazol.[34, 35] Cysts existing prior to treatment do not disappear but a profound reduction in the number of new cysts aspirated has been reported after 6 months treatment with a dose of 200 mg–400 mg a day. This effect seems to persist for some time after treatment has been stopped. Those patients who form multiple cysts should be offered the option of treatment with danazol. Some patients dislike taking regular tablets and many wish to persist by treatment with regular aspiration.

It has been suggested that withdrawal of caffeine and other methyl xanthines from the diet is also effective in reducing in the numbers of cysts aspirated from these patients.[43]

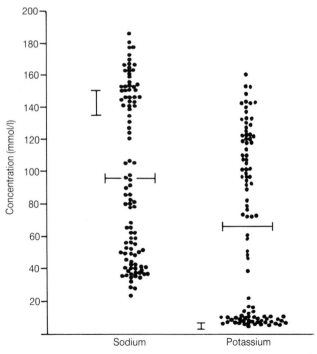

**Fig 5.3**  Values of sodium and potassium concentration in 100 samples of breast cyst fluid.

## Composition of cyst fluids

A variety of electrolytes, proteins and hormones have been measured in breast cyst fluids. Electrolyte concentrations have been shown to vary widely between individual cyst fluids.[28, 44, 45] This variation greatly exceeds that in plasma and the concentrations of sodium and potassium range from those of extracellular to those of intracellular fluid (Fig. 5.3). Attempts have been made to classify cyst fluids on the basis of these cations[28, 45-47] and two types of cysts have been defined (Fig. 5.4).[26, 28, 29] The two cyst groups separated on the basis of the sodium:potassium ratio appear to be lined by different types of epithelium, those with a sodium:potassium ratio < 3 being

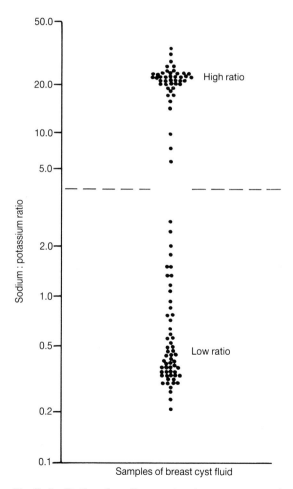

**Fig 5.4** Ratio of sodium:potassium concentration in 100 samples of breast cyst fluid.

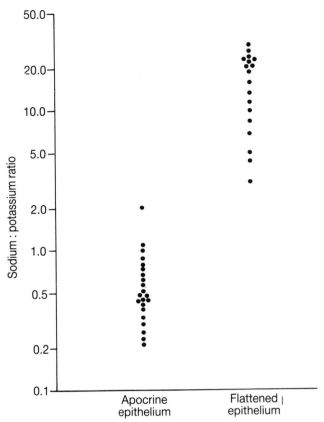

**Fig 5.5** Relationship between the nature of the epithelium lining breast cysts and the sodium:potassium content of the cyst fluid.

lined by apocrine epithelium and those with a sodium:potassium ratio $\geq 3$ being lined by flattened epithelium (Fig. 5.5).[26]

Numerous proteins in cyst fluid have been studied. The total protein content of these fluids tends to be less than that of plasma,[46] but specific proteins are found in concentrations greatly in excess of plasma concentrations. These specific proteins include carcinoembryonic antigen,[46, 48] a progesterone binding protein,[49] and a series of glycoproteins.[3] Immunoglobulins have also been quantified and characterised in cyst fluid. IgG is found in significantly higher concentrations in fluids with a high sodium:potassium ratio.[50] There is also a close correlation between the form of IgA and electrolyte composition, cyst fluids with a low sodium:potassium ratio containing predominantly the 11S form, with the 7S form being the major species in fluids with a high ratio.

The hormonal composition of cyst fluid has also been extensively investigated. Of the peptide hormones, growth Luteinising hormone, inteinising hormone, and follicle stimulating hormone are usually found in cyst fluid at lower concentrations than in plasma, whereas calcitonin, prolactin, and human chorionic gonadotrophin are present in greater amounts in cyst fluids.[36, 51] The unconjugated steroid hormones corticosterone, progesterone, testosterone, oestrone, and oestrodiol do not accumulate to any extent in cyst fluid. In contrast, androsterone, epiandrosterone, and dehydroepiandrosterone (DHA) and their conjugates do. For example, DHA sulphate may be present in cyst fluids in amounts many hundred times its plasma concentration (Fig. 5.6). There also appears to be a direct correlation between the concentration of these hormones and electrolyte composition

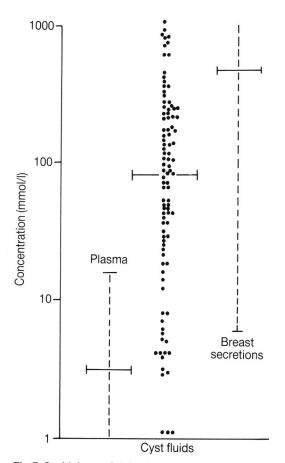

**Fig 5.6**  Values of dehydroepiandrosterone sulphate (DHA-S) in 100 samples of breast cyst fluid. (For comparison the ranges in plasma and breast secretions obtained by nipple aspiration have been added.) Horizontal bars represent median values.

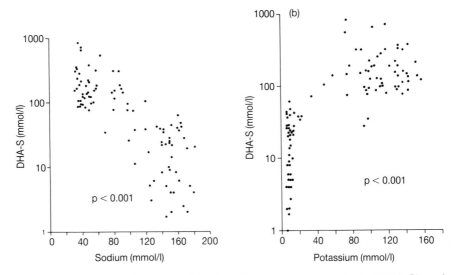

**Fig 5.7**  Correlation between dehydroepiandrosterone-sulphate (DHA-S) and
(a) sodium, and (b) potassium, in 100 cyst fluids.

(Fig. 5.7). It is of interest that the highest concentrations of DHA sulphate are
found in apocrine cysts, and that apocrine gland secretion from the axilla
also contains high amounts of this substance.[52] There is no correlation
between ionic composition and cyst size or colour.

Cyst fluid composition differs significantly from that of breast secretions
obtained from within the breast or from the nipple (Table 5.2). Cyst fluids
therefore cannot arise simply by a build up of breast secretions.

**Table 5.2**  Composition of plasma, breast secretions, and the two types of
breast cyst fluid

|  | Sodium : potassium ratio | DHA-S | Form of IgA |
|---|---|---|---|
| Plasma | High | → | 7S |
| Breast secretions: |  |  |  |
|   Deep | High | ↑ | 11S |
|   Nipple | High | ↑↑ | 11S |
| Breast cysts: |  |  |  |
|   Apocrine | Low | ↑↑ | 11S |
|   Flattened | High | −/↑ | 7S |

Deep secretions were obtained from the terminal ducts of mastectomy specimens for both
benign and malignant disease; nipple secretions were obtained by massage and suction.
DHAS – dehydroepiandrosterone sulphate.

## Microcysts

Despite there being two populations of macrocysts only a single population of microcysts have been identified. They all appear to be lined by apocrine epithelium and have an ionic and hormonal composition similar to apocrine macrocysts.[31] It is not known if these microcysts are the precursors of both populations of macrocysts.

## Natural history

There appears to be a difference in the natural history of the two cyst types. Patients with apocrine cysts (low sodium:potassium ratio) appear more likely to develop further cysts. (Table 5.3).

There is also a tendency for patients to develop cysts of the same type.[53] It is appreciated that some patients develop large numbers of cysts and as the number of cysts aspirated from any patient increases, so apparently does the likelihood that any cyst aspirated will be apocrine and thus contain fluid with a low sodium:potassium ratio (Fig. 5.8).

## Relationship of cystic disease to breast carcinoma

The published evidence relating cystic disease and breast carcinoma is conflicting and confusing. Most investigators have based their results on patients who have undergone breast biopsy, and use a histological definition of cystic disease. Since some of the histological features included in this definition are now considered part of normal breast involution,[32] the results from such studies may have little relevance to patients with clinically palpable breast cysts.

### Evidence relating cystic disease and breast cancer

*Epidemiological data*

Both cysts and cancer are more common in nulliparous women, suggesting a possible common aetiological factor.[1]

**Table 5.3** Relationship between cyst type at presentation and further or recurrent cyst formation

| Type of cyst at presentation | Number of patients | Number (%) developing further cysts |
|---|---|---|
| Apocrine (sodium:potassium $<3$) | 47 | 6(13) |
| Flattened (sodium:potassium $\geqslant 3$) | 47 | 34(72)* |
| Mixture of the two types | 6 | 3(50) |

* Significantly more patients with apocrine cysts developed further cysts than with flattened cysts ($p < 0.0005$).

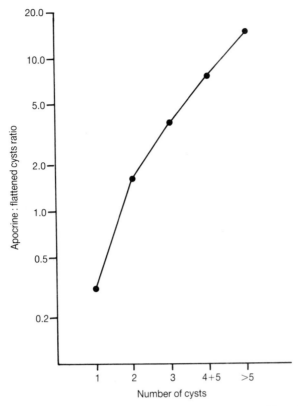

**Fig 5.8**   Ratio of apocrine: flattened cysts in 100 patients, with increasing total numbers of cysts aspirated over a two year follow up period.

*Frequency of cysts in patients with carcinoma*

Cooper[7] in 1829, when he first described cysts, noted that carcinoma could co-exist in the same breast, but early workers[11] considered these carcinomas to be incidental findings. Tietze in 1900[12] was the first to regard the 'adenomatous' proliferations seen in cystic breasts to be precancerous. It is difficult to find precise information as to the frequency of grossly visible cysts in breasts removed for carcinoma. The frequency of microscopic changes is usually recorded in publications relating so called cystic disease and breast cancer,[1, 3, 15, 54] but this does not help to define the relationship between clinically palpable cysts and breast cancer. Semb[15] found 27% of breasts with carcinoma contained visible cysts and, in a similar more detailed study, Foote and Stewart[54] found the same percentage of breasts with carcinoma had cysts greater than 1 mm in size. Haagensen[3] reported 7.6% of such breasts contained cysts greater than 2 mm in size and noted that

90% of patients whose breasts contained these cysts were under the age of 55. It is likely that few of these cysts were palpable and these studies are therefore of little value in determining whether clinical cystic disease is associated with an increased incidence of breast cancer. The fact that palpable cysts are not frequently found in breasts removed for carcinoma does not mean that the two diseases are unrelated. Cysts occur in a younger age group than breast cancer[3] and may have disappeared by the time a carcinoma arises.

## Frequency with which cystic disease precedes a breast carcinoma

Johnson in 1924[55] found only 2 patients of a series of 444 with breast cancer who had a history of previous breast cysts. Other studies, including those of Patey[56] and Foote and Stewart,[54] recorded a low incidence of cysts in patients with breast cancer. These studies were all performed prior to the introduction of treatment of cysts by simple aspiration, and definitions of what comprised cystic disease varied between these studies. Their relevance to modern practice is therefore open to doubt. It is likely that the true relationship of cystic disease and breast carcinoma can only be accurately determined by long term follow up studies.

A number of authors have attempted to conduct such studies. Most[5, 57-61] have reviewed series of patients undergoing biopsy for benign breast disease and performed a subsequent follow up to determine which histological features predicted an increased breast cancer risk. The problem with these studies is that they rely on patients who have undergone biopsy and do not identify those patients with palpable breast cysts. As most patients with palpable breast cysts do not undergo biopsy, the findings of these studies cannot be related directly to patients with clinical cystic disease. Similarly case control studies[62-67] have not identified patients with palpable cysts as a subgroup of those patients with so called 'cystic disease'. Page *et al*[60, 61] in their histological studies, did separate a group of patients with cysts which were likely to be palpable and showed no increased risk of subsequent malignancy in these patients. They did, however, show that patients with florid epithelial hyperplasia and atypia associated with cysts were at a significantly increased risk of breast cancer.[61]

## Follow up studies of patients with cystic disease treated by aspiration

Haagensen reported on 175 patients who developed breast carcinoma preceding or subsequent to cystic disease.[3, 68] The diagnosis of cystic disease was based either on biopsy or more frequently on cyst aspiration. The age distribution of these patients was similar to that of patients who did not have a history of cystic disease. The mean time from the diagnosis of cystic disease to the time of diagnosis of breast cancer was between 8 to 10 years.[68] From their data they calculated that the relative risk of developing breast cancer for patients with cystic disease was 2.48. (This comparison was with the expected number of breast cancers based on the state of Connecticut incidence rates by calendar year and age of the patient.) The relative risk

**Table 5.4** Patients with cystic disease and risk of subsequent breast carcinoma (from Haagensen et al[3])

| | | Number of cysts | |
|---|---|---|---|
| | Overall group | One | More than one |
| Number with cysts | 1808 | 978 | 830 |
| Number developing carcinoma | 124 | 58 | 66 |
| Number expected to develop carcinoma | 49.84 | 27.96 | 21.88 |
| Ratio observed: expected | 2:48 | 2:07 | 3:02 |

increased to 3.02 in patients who had more than one cyst (Table 5.4). There was no relationship between the age at which the patient developed her initial cyst and the cumulative probability of breast cancer.

The finding that cystic disease is associated with an increased incidence of breast cancer is supported by two other studies.[69, 70] Harrington and Lesnick[69] reported on 917 patients with cystic disease treated by aspiration, of whom 289 had at least a 5 year follow up. Nineteen of these 289 developed breast cancer, and 13 years after cyst aspiration they estimated 3.5 times more women had developed breast cancer than would have been expected. The average interval between initial cyst aspiration and the diagnosis of breast cancer was 7.9 years, remarkably similar to the 8 to 10 years of the Haagensen study. There was no increased incidence of breast carcinoma in the study by Harrington and Lesnick in those patients with multiple cysts. Jones and Bradbeer[70] in a similar follow up study of 332 patients with cystic disease also treated by aspiration, reported the subsequent incidence of carcinoma to be increased to 2.48 times that estimated from cancer registry data.

*Biochemical relationship between cystic disease and breast carcinoma*

Cyst fluid contains a variety of glycoproteins which are also present in breast carcinomas.[3] These glycoproteins may, however, simply be markers of apocrine epithelium. Cysts are frequently lined by apocrine epithelium, carcinoma can arise in such epithelium,[18, 22] and 10% of breast carcinomas show apocrine features.[71] The finding of a protein marker for such epithelium in cysts and breast cancer is therefore not surprising and does not imply a direct relationship between the two.

In conclusion, despite the large numbers of studies on this subject, the relationship between clinically palpable breast cystic disease and breast carcinoma is unclear. Further follow up studies of patients with cystic disease that has been treated by aspiration are required before it can be determined if these women are at any increased risk of breast cancer.

## Relationship of cyst type to breast cancer development and breast cancer risk

Insufficient data are available for firm conclusions to be drawn, but preliminary studies suggest that histological risk factors for malignancy may be more frequently seen in association with palpable apocrine cysts.[72] In a small series of patients with breast cancer and a history of cyst aspiration, the ratio of apocrine to flattened cysts was reported to be significantly higher than that found in the general population of patients with cysts.[72]

## References

1. Bonser GM, Dossett JA, Jull JW. *Human and Experimental Breast Cancer.* London, Pitman, 1961.
2. Azzopardi JG. *Problems in Breast Pathology.* London, WB Saunders, 1979.
3. Haagensen CD, Bodian C, Haagensen DE. *Breast carcinoma risk and detection.* Philadelphia, WB Saunders, 1981.
4. Frantz VK, Pickren JW, Melcher GW, Auchincloss H, Jr. Incidence of chronic cystic disease in so called 'normal breast'. *Cancer* 1951; **4**: 769–83.
5. Davis MM, Simons M, Davis JB. Cystic disease of the breast: relationship to carcinoma. *Cancer* 1964; **17**: 957–78.
6. Parks AG. The microanatomy of the breast. *Ann R Coll Surg Engl* 1959; **25**: 235–51.
7. Cooper AP. *Diseases of the Breast, Part 1.* London, Longmans, 1829.
8. Reclus P. La maladie kystique des mammelles. *Revue de chirurgie* 1883; **3**: 761–75.
9. Brissaud E. Anatomie pathologigue de la maladie kystique des mammelles. *Archives de physiologie normale et pathologique 1884*; **3**: 98–113.
10. Schimmelbusch C. Ueber das Cystadenom der wieblichen Milchdrüse. *Verhandlungen der Deutschen Gesellschaft für Chirurgie* 1890; **19**: 116–20.
11. König F. Mastitis chronica cystica. *Zentralblatt für Chirurgie* 1893; **20**: 49–53.
12. Tietze F. Ueber das cystadenoma mammae (Schimmelbusch) und seine beziehungen zum carcinom der Brustdrüse. *Deutsche Zeitschrift für Chirurgie* 1900; **56**: 512–48.
13. Bloodgood JC. Senile parenchymatous hypertrophy of the female breast: its relation to cyst formation and carcinoma. *Surg Gynecol Obstet* 1906; **3**: 721–30.
14. McFarland M. Residual lactational acini in the female breast: their relation to chronic cystic mastitis and malignant disease. *Arch Surg* 1922; **5**: 1–64.
15. Semb C. Pathologico-anatomical and clinical investigations of fibro-adenomatosis cystica mammae and its relation to other pathological conditions in mamma especially cancer. *Acta Chir Scand* 1928; **64** (suppl x): 1–484.
16. Creighton C. *Cancers and other Tumours of the Breast.* London, Williams and Norgate, 1902.
17. Nicholson GW. Studies in tumour formation. *Guy's Hospital Report* 1923; **73**: 37.
18. Ewing J. *Neoplastic diseases.* 4th ed. Philadelphia, WB Saunders, 1940.
19. Krompecher E. Über Schweissdrüssenzysten der Brustdrüse und deren krebse. *Verhandlungen der Deutschen Pathologischen Gesellschaft* 1913; **16**: 365–84.
20. Von Saar GF. Ueber cystadenoma mammae und mastitis chronica cystica. *Achiv für Klinische Chirurgie* 1907; **84**: 223–79.

21. Cheatle GL, Cutler M. *Tumours of the Breast*. London, Arnold, 1931.
22. Dawson EK. Sweat gland carcinoma of the breast. *Edinburgh Medical Journal* 1932; **39**: 409–38.
23. Lendrum AC. On the pink epithelium of the cystic breast and the staining of the granules. *Journal of Pathology and Bacteriology* 1945; **57**: 267–70.
24. Wellings SR, Jensen HM, Marcum RG. An atlas of subgross pathology of the human breast with reference to possible precancerous lesions. *JNCI* 1975; **55**: 231–73.
25. Wellings SR. Development of human breast cancer. *Adv Cancer Res* 1980; **31**: 287–314.
26. Dixon JM, Miller WR, Scott WN, Forrest APM. The morphological basis of human breast cyst populations *Br J Surg* 1983; **70**: 604–6.
27. Miller WR, Humeniuk V, Kelly RW. Dehydroepiandrosterone sulphate in breast secretions. *J Steroid Biochem* 1980; **13**: 145–51.
28. Miller WR, Dixon JM, Scott WN, Forrest APM. Classification of human breast cysts according to electrolyte and androgen conjugate composition. *Clinical Oncology* 1983; **9**: 227–32.
29. Dixon JM. *A Study of Androgen Conjugates and Apocrine Differentiation in the Human Breast*. MD Thesis, University of Edinburgh, 1984, pp 55–172.
30. Schwartz GF. Cystic disease, a definition. In: Angeli, A, Bradlow HL, Dogliotti L. (Eds) *Endocrinology of Cystic Breast Disease*. New York, Raven Press, 1983, pp 1–6.
31. Dixon JM, Scott WN, Miller WR. An analysis of the content and morphology of human breast microcysts. *Eur J Surg Oncol* 1985; **11**: 151–4.
32. Hughes LE, Mansel RE, Webster DJT. Aberrations of normal development and involution (ANDI): A new perspective on pathogenesis and nomenclature of benign breast disorders. *Lancet* 1987; **ii**: 1316–9.
33. Angeli A, Dogliotti L. Fibrocystic disease of the breast. A re-visit and new perspectives. Amsterdam, Excerpta Medica, 1984.
34. Rasmussen T, Tobiassen T, Doberl A. Reduction of cysts in fibrocystic breast disease during and after Danazol treatment. *Ann NY Acad Sci* 1986; **464**: 622–5.
35. Hinton CP, Dowle C, Locker A, *et al.* Modification of the natural history of cystic disease of the breast by a short course of danazol: evidence from a controlled trial. *Br J Clin Pract* 1982; **42** (suppl 56): 56–57.
36. Melis GB, Guarnieri G, Paoletti AM, *et al.* Clinical significance of hormonal evalution in peripheral blood and in breast cyst fluid of women with benign breast disease. In: Angeli A, Bradlow HL, Dogliotti L. (Eds) *Endocrinology of Cystic Breast Disease*. New York, Raven Press, 1983, pp 101–12.
37. Mauvais-Jarvis P, Sitruk-Ware R, Kutten F, Sterkers N. Luteal phase insufficiency: a common pathophysiological factor in development of benign and malignant breast disease. In: Bulbrook RD, Taylor DJ. (Eds) *Commentaries on Research in Breast Disease*. New York, Alan J Liss, 1979, pp 25–9.
38. Miller WR, Forrest APM. Androgen conjugates in human breast secretions and cyst fluids. In: Angeli A, Bradlow HL, Dogliotti L. (Eds) *Endocrinology of Cystic Breast Disease*. New York, Raven Press, 1983, pp 77–84.
39. Cowen PN, Benson EA. Cytological study of fluid from breast cysts. *Br J Surg* 1979; **66**: 209–11.
40. Forrest APM, Kirkpatrick JR, Roberts MM. Needle aspiration of breast cysts. *Br Med J* 1975; **iii**: 30–1.
41. Kalisher L. Intracystic carcinoma of the breast. *Breast* 1977; **30**: 32–3.
42. Dixon JM, Clarke PJ. Refilling of breast cysts as an indication for breast biopsy. *Lancet* 1985; **ii**: 608.
43. Minton JP, Abou-Isa H, Reiches N, Roseman JM. Clinical and biochemical

studies on methylxanthine-related fibrocystic breast disease. *Surgery* 1981; **90**: 229-304.

44. Gatzy JT, Zayloun MP, Gaskins K, Pearlmann WH. Electrolytes in breast cyst fluid. *Clin Chem* 1979; **25**: 745-8.
45. Bradlow HL, Skidmore FD, Schwartz MK, Fleisher M. Cation levels in human breast cyst fluids. *Clinical Oncology* 1981; **7**: 388-90.
46. Gairard B, Gros CM, Koehl C, Renaud R. Proteins and ionic components in breast cyst fluids. In :Angeli A, Bradlow HL, Dogliotti L. (Eds) *Endocrinology of Cystic Breast Disease*. New York, Raven Press, 1983, pp 191-6.
47. Orlandi F, Bocuzzi G, Corradin MP, *et al*. Cations and dehydroisoandrosterone – sulphate in human breast cyst fluid. *Ann NY Acad Sci* 1986; **464**: 596-98.
48. Fleisher M, Oettgen HF, Breed CN, *et al*. CEA like material in fluid from benign cysts of the breast *Clin Chem* 1974; **20**: 41-42.
49. Pearlman WH, Gueriguian JD, Sawyer ME. A specific progesterone-binding component of human breast cyst fluid. *J Biol Chem* 1973; **248**: 5736-41.
50. Dixon JM, Miller WR, Yap PL, *et al*. Further studies on human breast cyst fluids. *Br J Surg* 1983; **70**: 684.
51. Bradlow HL, Schwartz MK, Fleisher M, *et al*. Hormone levels in human breast cyst fluids. In: Angeli A, Bradlow HL, Dogliotti L. (Eds) *Endocrinology of Cystic Breast Disease*. New York, Raven Press, 1983, pp 59-75.
52. Labows JN, Preti G, Hoelzle E, *et al*. Steroid analysis of human apocrine secretion. *Steroids* 1979; **34**: 249-98.
53. Dixon JM, Scott WN, Miller WR. Natural history of cystic disease; importance of cyst type. *Br J Surg* 1985; **72**: 190-92.
54. Foote FW, Stewart FW. Comparative studies of cancerous and non cancerous breasts. *Ann Surg* 1945; **121**: 6-53.
55. Johnson R. Some clinical aspects of carcinoma of the breast. *Br J Surg* 1924/25; **12**: 630-32.
56. Patey DH. Chronic cystic mastitis and carcinoma; collective review. *Int Abstr Surg* 1939; **68**: 575-78.
57. Warren S. The relation of 'chronic mastitis' to carcinoma of the breast. *Surg Gynecol Obstet* 1940; **71**: 257-73.
58. Veronesi U, Pizzocaro F. Breast cancer in women subsequent to cystic disease of the breast. *Surg Gynecol Obstet* 1968; **126**: 529-32.
59. Monson RR, Yen S, MacMahon B, Warren S. Chronic mastitis and carcinoma of the breast. *Lancet* 1976; **ii**: 224-26.
60. Page DL, Vander Zwag R, Rogers LW, *et al*. Relation between component parts of fibrocystic disease complex and breast cancer. *JNCI* 1978; **61**: 1055-63.
61. Dupont WD, Page DL. Risk factors for breast cancer in women with proliferative breast disease. *N Engl J Med* 1985; **312**: 146-51.
62. Roberts MM, Jones V, Elton RA, *et al*. Risk of breast cancer in women with a history of benign disease of the breast. *Br Med J* 1984; **288**: 275-78.
63. Duffy SW, Roberts MM, Elton RA. Risk factors for breast cancer: relevance to screening. *J Epidemiol Community Health* 1983; **37**: 127-31.
64. Shapiro S, Strax P, Venet L, Fink R. The search for risk factors in breast cancer. *Am J Public Health* 1968; **58**: 820-35.
65. Vessey MP, Doll R, Jones K. An epidemiological study of oral contraceptives and breast cancer. *Br Med J* 1979; **i**: 941-44.
66. Wynder EL, MacCormack FA, Stellman SD. The epidemiology of breast cancer in 785 US caucasian women. *Cancer* 1978; **41**: 2341-45.
67. Brinton LA, Williams RR, Hoover RN. Breast cancer risk factors among screening program participants. *JNCI* 1979; **62**: 37-44.

68. Haagensen CD. *Disease of the breast*. 2nd ed. Philadelphia, WB Saunders, 1971.
69. Harrington E, Lesnik G. The association between gross cysts of the breast and breast cancer. *Breast* 1981; **7**: 113–17.
70. Jones BM, Bradbeer JW. The presentation and progress of macroscopic breast cysts. *Br J Surg* 1980; **67**: 669–71.
71. Miller WR, Telford J, Dixon JM, Shivas AA. Androgen metabolism and apocrine differentiation in human breast cancer. *Breast Cancer Res Treat* 1985; **5**: 67–73.
72. Dixon JM, Lumsden AB, Miller WR. The relationship of cyst type to risk factors for breast cancer and subsequent development of breast cancer. *Eur J Cancer Clin Oncol* 1985; **21**: 1047–50.

# 6

# Nipple discharge

U CHETTY

## Introduction

In most non-lactating women a small quantity of fluid can be expressed from the ducts of the nipple if a negative pressure is applied[1, 2] or if enough circum-areolar pressure with the fingers is supplied.

Spontaneous nipple discharges must be regarded as abnormal although in most cases the aetiology is benign. As a reason for specialist referral this makes up less than 5% of new patients in a breast clinic. In Haagenson's series[3] up until 1978 this figure was 1.8% and in a recent survey from the Edinburgh clinic, of 5000 new patients 4.8% complained primarily of discharge. Incidence figures can be misleading and are not always comparable; for example the Edinburgh figure was taken from a detailed questionnaire, but a substantial proportion (33%) failed to produce a discharge on subsequent examination. In contrast, all Haagenson's cases complained of, and produced, a discharge; this probably accounts for the lower incidence figure which must have discounted those referrals in whom the diagnosis could not be confirmed. Even allowing for differing definitions of nipple discharge, it is nevertheless an uncommon problem.

## Aetiology and classification

Much of the confusion over correct management of nipple discharge arises from misleading data, most of which are historical and refer to patterns of disease presentation not seen today. Early series[4] reported a high incidence of associated or causative cancer, often over 50%, but in most cases a coexistent mass was found. Because of this and the uncertainty of cancer risks associated with benign pathology, mastectomy for solitary papilloma was commonly performed into the 1950s at the Mayo clinic.[5] It is the experience of most surgeons today that nipple discharge is uncommonly related to cancer or cancer risk but contemporary, hard scientific data to support this are hard to find. When spontaneous discharges of all sorts are reported as in the Edinburgh survey the principal causes in 265 cases were: duct ectasia (27%); duct papilloma (10%); carcinoma (5%); galactorrhoea (3%) and no abnormality (33%).

A large series on single duct nipple discharge has recently been reported from Nottingham[6] and their results are summarised in Table 6.1; only 7% had cancer and all were *in situ* lesions. Whatever the source of information the most common causes for discharge are duct ectasia and duct papilloma, with early or *in situ* ductal carcinoma making only a small proportion.

**Table 6.1**   Causes of single duct nipple discharge in 170 patients (Nottingham 1988)

| Diagnosis | Number (%) |
| --- | --- |
| Duct papilloma | 77 (45) |
| Benign disease (for example, duct ectasia) | 80 (47) |
| Cancer *in situ* | 12  (7) |
| No abnormality | 1  (0.6) |

## Classification

Nipple discharges can be conveniently classified into those caused by factors outside the breast (Table 6.2), which are predominantly neuroendocrine, those related to disease of the nipple areola complex and – by far the most common – those related to the ductal system (Table 6.3).

## Nipple discharge without primary breast disease (Table 6.2)

Prolonged use of the oral contraceptive pill is occasionally associated with a slight serous or milky discharge which is bilateral. Paradoxically this may also develop temporarily when oral contraceptive pills are stopped.

If the pill is being taken it could be stopped, or the discharge ignored. Other drugs known to be associated with a discharge (usually milky) include the phenothiazines, reserpine, methyldopa, tricyclic antidepressants, cimetidine, and haloperidol.

**Table 6.2**   Nipple discharge due to causes outside the breast

1. Longterm oral contraceptive usage (bilateral, not bloody)
2. Middle and last trimester of pregnancy (bilateral, bloody)
3. Pubescent girls during maximal breast enlargement (bilateral, serous)
4. Squeezing of breast and nipples (galactorrhoea)
5. Post chest trauma (galactorrhoea)
6. Pituitary disease (galactorrhoea)
7. Hypothyroidism (galactorrhoea)
8. Drugs (variable)

There are several instances, perhaps 'physiological' but rare, in which discharges can cause great concern; firstly the bilateral serous discharge which accompanies menstruation at the time of puberty when there is a concomitant rapid development of the breasts and, secondly, the bilateral blood stained discharge of pregnant women in the middle and last trimester. These are innocent and resolve when the physiological event has passed.

Repeated squeezing of the nipple or periareolar area will also induce a milky discharge and whether by over enthusiam in self examination, or love play, should be discouraged. If continued repeatedly full lactation can be induced. Severe trauma to the chest – for example, thoracoplasty and pneumonectomy – has also been reported to induce temporary lactation although the mechanism is unknown.[7]

Both bronchogenic carcinoma and hypernephroma have rarely been associated with discharge and probably by tumorogenic hormone activity.

*Galactorrhoea*

Galactorrhoea can be defined as an inappropriate and persistent white milky discharge from the nipple, usually arising from multiple ducts and often bilateral. In a study of 235 patients with galactorrhoea, Kleinberg *et al*[8] showed that 20% of all patients and 34% with associated amenorrhoea had radiologically evident pituitary tumours; these patients had the highest serum prolactin concentrations. The largest single group (32%) consisted of women with idiopathic galactorrhoea without amenorrhoea; prolactins were normal in 86% of these. Other causes include idiopathic galactorrhoea with amenorrhoea (8.5%); Chiari-Frommel syndrome (7.6%), tranquilising drugs (6.8%), cessation of the oral contraceptive pill (5.1%); hypothyroidism (4.2%), and the empty sella syndrome (2%).

The serum prolactin concentration should be routinely measured in all cases. Unfortunately there is no consensus on the upper limit of normal – Jeffcoate and colleagues[9] suggest that a prolactin concentration of less than 700 mU/L virtually excludes important disease in women, whereas a value between 700 and 1000 mU/L is only of doubtful pathological significance.

In patients with large pituitary tumours and hyperprolactinaemia, it is not always clear whether the high prolactin occurs because the tumour itself is secreting prolactin or because of compression of the pituitary stalk by non-functioning tumour, thus preventing transmission of the hypothalamic prolactin inhibitory factor, dopamine, into the anterior pituitary.

Bevan *et al*[10] found that patients with a serum prolactin concentration of less than 3000 mU/L were likely to have a non-functioning tumour whereas those with concentrations greater than 8000 mU/L were almost certain to have a prolactinoma. Between the two limits, either disease was possible.

It is usual to undertake a computed tomogram of the pituitary in someone whose serum prolactin is raised. The demonstration of a macroadenoma is an indication for treatment either by surgery or radiotherapy. The importance of a microadenoma is much less clear because about 40% of normal premenopausal women have been shown to have these on computed tomography.[11] Patients who are hyperprolactinaemic, have symptoms, and whose tomogram excludes a macroadenoma can be treated with bromocryptine.

All the above states are related to a systemic 'fault' and cause 'bilateral' discharges; this feature alone in the history strongly mitigates against serious primary disease of the breast.

## Nipple discharge caused by disease of the nipple areola complex (Table 6.3)

This is generally an uncommon cause of discharge or crusting but is nevertheless important as unnecessary investigations may be saved.

### Nipple adenoma

A nipple adenoma is rare but easy to diagnose. It usually presents with a blood stained discharge or change in colour of the nipple skin to red. Occasionally an ulcer develops. Examination reveals an indiscrete mass in the substance of the superficial layer of the nipple. It is difficult or even impossible to exclude Paget's disease, and diagnosis rests with histology having excised a small wedge of the abnormal epithelium under local anaesthetic. With the diagnosis of adenoma established, definitive treatment depends on the extent of the lesion. In many, total excision of the nipple will be required but, if not, extensive local excision with conservation of the nipple is possible.[12] There is no evidence that nipple adenoma predisposes to carcinoma.

### Nipple eczema and the more common Paget's disease of the nipple

These can conveniently be discussed together. Eczema or dermatitis can effect the nipple like any other area of skin; it is usually caused by irritation from clothes or cosmetics and may become secondarily infected with skin organisms. There are several features in the history and examination which help the clinician distinguish between the two. Firstly, Paget's disease does not quickly spread throughout the nipple areola complex: this is certainly a feature of eczema which frequently appears and spreads to most of the complex within a few weeks. Secondly, eczema never destroys the nipple, but Paget's can. Finally, it is almost unheard of for eczema to affect only the nipple and not the areola and, conversely, for Paget's to affect the areola without the nipple. Whatever the clinical impression, diagnosis can only be made by wedge excision under local anaesthesia; trials of steroid creams must be discouraged where eczema is suspected unless they take place under controlled conditions with prolonged follow up. The place of cytology from scrapings has yet to be formally assessed but this may be a quick and convenient method of diagnosis if 'positive.' It should be disregarded if negative. Similarly a mammogram may show the small areas of calcification of association retroareola intraduct carcinoma but should not be relied upon for diagnosis.

The treatment of eczema when confirmed is to remove any related aggravating factors and treat if necessary with a short course of topical steroid. If any superadded infection is suspected than a swab should be taken and the appropriate antibiotic prescribed. The treatment of Paget's disease is beyond the scope of this chapter but the choice for many is simple mastectomy. This condition is certainly not as 'benign' as often suggested, as most large series with long follow up show a mortality of 20% with skin lesions alone, but 50% if there is any associated palpable lump.[13]

**Table 6.3** Nipple discharge due to causes within the breast

| Nipple: areola complex | Ductal: |
|---|---|
| 1. Nipple adenoma | 1. Duct papilloma (s) |
| 2. Eczema | 2. Duct ectasia |
| 3. Pagets disease | 3. Cancer *in situ*, or early invasive ductal cancer |
| 4. Ulcerating carcinoma | 4. Cystic disease |
| 5. Inversion of nipple and maceration | 5. Idiopathic |

*Long-standing inversion of the nipple associated with maceration*

This is rare, but seen most often in elderly people. The inverted nipple forms a cavity which is rarely cleaned and the lining epithelium gradually becomes macerated. The injured skin itself produces a discharge but this may occasionally be associated with the irritative effects of discharge from ectatic ducts. Whatever the cause, the condition is easily resolved by everting the nipple and regular cleaning; it is easy to distinguish from Paget's disease, but if any doubt exists biopsy should always be performed.

## Nipple discharge caused by disease of the ductal system (Table 6.3)

Of the several conditions commonly associated with nipple discharge most are caused by ductal disease. Of these duct ectasia and duct papilloma are by far the most common but *in situ* ductal or early invasive cancer are the most important. These will be discussed in some detail, and cystic disease has been dealt with in *chapter 5*.

*Duct ectasia*
*Terminology* – Duct ectasia is a benign disease complex of unknown aetiology in which duct dilatation is a major feature.[14] Various other terms have been used to describe this condition, each based on one of the many clinical or pathological features the particular author considered important.

Inflammation around the large and medium sized ducts, a histological landmark of this condition, is known as periductal mastitis.[15] The term 'plasma cell mastitis' draws attention to the fact that plasma cells are frequently found in the chronic inflammatory cell infiltrate around the ducts. The presence of pasty inspissated intraductal material gave rise to the diagnostic phrase comedomastitis.[16] The term 'obliterative mastitis' has been applied to the late stage of this disease, when there is total obliteration of the ductal lumen by fibrous tissue with complete disappearance of the epithelial lining.[17, 18]

Page and Anderson[19] suggest that the term 'duct ectasia' be maintained until a pathogenetically or aetiologically related phrase is suggested to replace it.

*Pathogenesis and aetiology* of this condition remain controversial. Earlier workers regarded ductal dilatation with stasis of ductal contents as the initial manifestation of the disorder, with periductal inflammation a secondary phenomenon. The fact that inflammatory cases of the disease predominate in the younger age group suggests that periductal inflammation may be the primary abnormality and that duct dilatation is secondary to this.[20, 21]

A possible role for developmentally inverted nipples in the aetiology of this condition has been suggested by Rees *et al*,[22] though it is more likely that the retracted nipple associated with it is the result rather than the cause.[15]

More recently it has been suggested that anaerobic bacteria have a role in the pathogenesis of periductal mastitis. A study in which bacteriological swabs of nipple discharge or pus were immediately inoculated into transport medium (Robertson's cooked meat broth) showed that bacteria could be isolated in 27% of patients with uncomplicated duct ectasia, 83% of patients with an associated inflammatory mass, and all patients with either a non-lactating breast abscess or mamillary fistula.[23] It is unlikely that anaerobic infection is a primary cause of this condition but more probable that bacterial infection develops secondary to stasis in large ducts and that many of the secondary complications (mamillary fistula, non-lactation abscess, and inflammatory mass) are manifestations of this infection.[24]

*Incidence* – Azzopardi reported the changes of duct ectasia in 30–40% of surgical and necropsy specimens of women above the age of 50 years. In a post mortem study Sanderson[25] found duct ectasia as an incidental finding in 25% of women of all ages. The clinical manifestations of the conditions are, however, much less common.

*Clinical features and treatment* – Nipple discharge is the most common symptom of duct ectasia. It is usually bilateral and arises from multiple ducts. The discharge may be straw, green, or brown in colour and often of paste-like consistency – it is not usually blood stained but is often positive for haemoglobin on dipstick testing (Ames) particularly after enthusiastic manoeuvres to express it.

Affected patients are invariably postmenopausal and usually present because the discharge is embarrassing or offensive and for reassurance that there is no sinister disease. Apart from the expression of discharge at the nipple from multiple ducts in one or both breasts there is no abnormal finding. The only investigation worth performing is a biplanar mammogram to exclude a coexistent carcinoma.

Further treatment depends upon the individual patient. Most are happy to live with their leaky ducts once the spectre of malignant disease has been removed. For those whose discharge is unacceptable the only treatment is surgery and the procedure of choice is a retroareolar excision of ducts (*chapter 3*). This removes the retroareolar major duct complex and allows any nipple inversion to be corrected. The only serious long standing complication is that of reduced nipple sensation, but this can be avoided by an infra-areolar incision, entering the correct plane and avoiding too superficial a dissection.

The complications of duct ectasia (Fig. 6.1), those of periareolar inflammation, abscess, and fistula formation, are serious causes of morbidity they are dealt with in *chapter 7*.

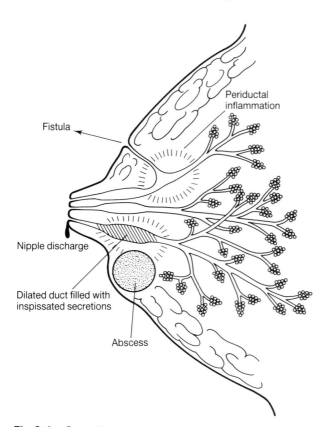

**Fig 6.1**   Complications of duct ectasia.

*Duct papilloma*

*Terminology* – Some confusion has arisen, as the term papilloma has been used to describe two anatomically different conditions. The lactiferous sinus and adjacent large ducts are affected by the 'true' or 'central' papilloma which is usually solitary, confined to large ducts of the subareola area, and often presents with nipple discharge. The peripheral variety of papilloma originates within lobular units and extends along small ducts. It is usually multifocal and related to epithelial hyperplasia.[26]

*Histology* – The central papilloma is a true papilloma with epithelium covered arborescent fronds of fibrovascular stroma and attached to the wall of the duct by a stalk. The covering epithelium is usually of the normal two cell population (that is, cuboidal or columnar epithelium and myoepithelial cells).

*Association with cancer* – The solitary papilloma is not thought to be premalignant by most pathologists.[27] Neither Haagenson *et al*[28] nor Carter[29] found in careful follow up studies of such women that carcinoma developed subsequently to a significant degree.

Multiple peripheral papillomas are associated with an increased risk of developing breast cancer[28] but this is probably because of the epithelial hyperplasia and atypia associated with this condition rather than the papilloma *per se*.[19]

*Clinical presentation and management* – Both central and more peripheral papillomas present with a discharge from a single duct of the nipple which may be serous or frankly bloodstained. The presence of blood, either frank or microscopic, confers no discriminating value on the likely cause. A lump may be felt at examination (in about one third of cases) and management then continues as for any discrete mass. Careful examination of the periareolar region may reveal a point, pressure on which causes the discharge to gush out of the duct. Occasionally the papilloma is close to the duct orifice and can be seen as it prolapses out of the ostium.

Cytology of single or unilateral nipple discharges is worthwhile if expert cytology is available, but results are not nearly as good as with aspiration cytology of solid lesions, and should be treated with caution. Knight *et al* in 1986[30] presented a series of 114 cases of nipple discharge with cytology, and 100 failed to provide an adequate cellular smear. Only five of the 10 related carcinomas were identified. Similar difficulties were found by the Japanese in a large series from Tokyo;[31] it was noted that cells in the discharge were frequently shrunken and difficult to identify. Like cytology of other organs, a definite diagnosis of carcinoma is invariably reliable but negative results should be regarded with caution. Cytology alone cannot diagnose duct papilloma.

Ductography has few exponents in this country and most centres only use it in exceptional circumstances. A recent large series was reported from Huddersfield; of 89 single nipple discharges, 12 malignant lesions over 5 cm from the nipple were found and all individual papillomas identified.[32] Most surgeons would have operated on these anyway, thus questioning the management value of the investigation.

The treatment of choice for either central or more peripheral papilloma is microdochectomy. This is described in detail in *chapter 11*. After cannulating the duct from which the discharge can be expressed, the duct and segment which drains is then completely excised. This can be achieved through either a radial incision or a more cosmetic periareolar incision, though this may lead to some loss of sensation.

A recent study from Nottingham[6] suggests an expectant policy with single duct discharge and normal mammograms. Their conclusion is based on a review of 98 consecutive patients undergoing microdochectomy in which a total of 8 patients were found to have ductal carcinoma *in situ*, 6 of whom had abnormal mammograms. A proportion of patients will undoubtedly prefer surgical exploration and an end to the problem; it remains to be seen what happens to papillomas if left untreated.

*Early or* in situ *ductal carcinoma*

A detailed discussion of nipple discharge in relation to invasive carcinoma is inappropriate in this chapter, but brief mention will be made to its more frequent association with *in situ* disease. In most contemporary series, *in situ* ductal carcinoma is responsible for between 5 and 10% of unilateral nipple discharge. This may be either serous or blood stained but confers no prognostic significance.

Nipple discharge alone or in association with a mass or Paget's disease were presenting clinical features in about one third of unscreened *in situ* ductal cancers in a recent series.[33] *In situ* ductal disease presenting with discharge in this series did not correlate with multifocality or histological type. There are scanty data about how often there is a suspicious mammographic abnormality but in the Nottingham series[6] 6 of 8 *in situ* tumours producing discharge were diagnosed on mammography.

The optimum treatment of *in situ* disease after biopsy confirmation is unknown, and it will take long term studies to establish this. Paradoxically it may be that mastectomy is indicated for most of these cases, particularly where disease is extensive and multifocal. How adjuvant hormone therapy and radiotherapy may alter the course of non-invasive disease are also important questions to be answered.

## Management of nipple discharge in the clinic

When presented with a patient complaining of nipple discharge it is helpful to have a scheme or algorithm of management (Fig. 6.2). To some extent this must vary according to local expertise but of great value after clinical assessment is a high quality biplanar mammogram. Cytology of discharge fluids and ductography are ignored in this plan as they are seldom available and of uncertain value. In patients with galactorrhoea of no obvious cause, referral to an endocrinologist should be considered.

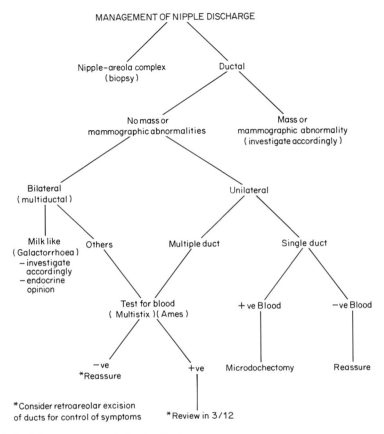

**Fig 6.2**   Management of nipple discharge.

# References

1. Petrakis NL, Mason L, Lee R, *et al.* Association of race, age, menopausal status and serum type with breast fluid secretion in non-lactating women as determined by nipple aspiration. *JNCI* 1975; **54**: 829–23.
2. Miller WR, Anderson TJ. Oestrogen, progesterone and the breast. In: Studd JW, Whitehead MJ. (Eds) *The Menopause.* Oxford, Blackwell Scientific Publications, 1988, pp 234–46.
3. Haagenson CD. *Diseases of the Breast.* 3rd ed. Philadelphia, WB Saunders, 1986, pp 138.
4. Adair FE. Sanguinous discharge from the nipple and its significance in relation to cancer of the breast. *Ann Surg* 1930; **91**: 197.
5. Madalin HE, Clayett OT, Macdonald JR. Lesions of the breast associated with discharge from the nipple. *Ann Surg* 1957; **146**: 751.
6. Locker AP, Salea MH, Ellis IO, *et al.* Microdochectomy for single-duct discharge from the nipple. *Br J Surg* 1988; **75**: 700–2.
7. Salkin D, Dains EW. Lactation following thoracoplasty and pneumonectomy. *Journal of Thoracic Surgery* 1949; **18**: 580.

8. Kleinberg DL, Noll GL, Frantz AG. Glactorrhoea: a study of 235 cases, including 48 with Pituitary Tumours. *N Engl J Med* 1977; **296**: 589–600.
9. Jeffcoate SC, Bacon RRA, Beestall GN, et al. Assay for prolactin: guidelines for the provision of a clinical biochemistry service *Am Clin Biochem* 1986; **23**: 638–51.
10. Bevan JS, Burke CW, Esiri MM, Adams CBI. Misinterpretation of prolactin levels leading to management errors in patients with sella enlargement. *Am J Med* 1987; **82**: 29–32.
11. Editorial. Hyperprolactinaemia: when is a prolactinoma not a prolactinoma? *Lancet* 1987; **ii**: 1002–4.
12. Haagenson CD. *Diseases of the Breast*. 3rd ed. Philadelphia, WB Saunders, 1986, pp 173.
13. Haagenson CD. *Diseases of the Breast*. 3rd ed. Philadelphia, WB Saunders, 1986, pp 778.
14. Haagenson CD. *Diseases of the Breast*. 2nd ed. Philadelphia, WB Saunders, pp 185–89.
15. Azzopardi JG. *Problems in Breast Pathology*. Philadelphia, WB Saunders, 1979.
16. Tice GI, Dockerty MB, Harrington SW. Comedomastitis, a clinical and pathological study of data in 172 cases. *Surg Gynecol Obstet* 1948; **87**: 525–40.
17. Ingier A. Uber obliterierendo mastitis. *Virchows Archive für Pathologische Anatomie und Physiologie für Klinische Medizin*. 1909; **198**: 338–45.
18. Payne RL, Strauss AF, Glasser RD. Mastitis Obliterans. *Surgery* 1943; **14**: 719–27.
19. Page DL, Anderson TJ. In: *Diagnostic Histopathology of the Breast*. Edinburgh, Churchill Livingstone, 1987, pp
20. Bonser GM, Dossett JA, Jull JW. *Human and Experimental Breast Cancer*. London, Pitman Medical, 1961.
21. Dixon JM, Anderson TJ, Lumsden AB, et al. Mammary duct ectasia. *Br J Surg* 1983; **70**: 601–3.
22. Rees BI, Gravelle IH, Hughes LE. Nipple retraction in duct ectasia. *Br J Surg* 1977; **64**: 577–80.
23. Bundred NJ, Dixon MJ, Lumsden AB, et al. Are the lesions of duct ectasia sterile? *Br J Surg* 1985; **72**: 844–45.
24 Browning J, Bigrigg A, Taylor I. *J R Soc Med* 1986; **79**: 715–16.
25. Sandison AT. *An Autopsy Study of the Adult Human Breast*. National Cancer Institute Monograph No 8. Washington DC: US Department of Health Education Medicine, 1982, pp 1–45.
26. Ohuchi N, Abe R, Takahashi T, Tezuka F. Origins and extension of interductal papillomas of the breast – a three-dimensional reconstruction study. *Breast Cancer Res Treat* 1984; **4**: 117–218.
27. Page DL, Anderson T. In: *Diagnostic Histopathology of the Breast*. Edinburgh, Churchill Livingstone, 1987.
28. Haagenson CD, Bodians C, Haagenson DE. *Breast Carcinoma Risk and Detection*. Philadelphia, WB Saunders, pp 146–237.
29. Carter D. Intraductal papillary tumours of the breast: a study of 78 cases. *Cancer* 1977; **39**: 1689–92.
30. Knight D, Lowell D, Heimann A, Dunne E. Aspiration of the breast and nipple discharge cytology. *Surg Gynecol Obstet* 1986; **163**: 415–20.
31. Uci Y, Wanatabe Y, Hirota T, et al. Cytologic diagnosis of breast carcinoma with nipple discharge. *Acta Cytol* 1980; **24**: 522–28.
32. Harris WG. Ductograph for nipple discharge. *Lancet* 1984; **i**: 110.
33. Fentiman IS, Fagg N, Millis RR, Hayward JL. *In situ* carcinoma of the breast: implications of disease pattern and treatment. *Eur J Surg Oncol* 1986; 261–66.

# 7

# Breast abcesses and problems with lactation

K ROGERS

## Breast abscesses

There are a number of conditions embraced by the term 'mastitis' which are unrelated to true breast abscesses which, by definition, contain pus. Of these, neonatal mastitis caused by persistence of maternal hormones, and pubertal mastitis caused by a relative imbalance of male and female hormones, are never associated with acute inflammation or suppuration. Similarly the 'mastitis' known more accurately as cyclical mastalgia is never associated with inflammation and is probably a consequence of subtle endocrine aberration.

If one excludes the rare abscess due to chronic inflammatory conditions – for example, tuberculosis, syphilis, and actinomycosis – breast abscesses are divided into those associated with lactation and others non-lactational; the latter group will be discussed in the following section. Non-lactational breast abscesses are conveniently divided into peripheral abscesses (which arise in the outer part of the breast) and those that arise from the large ducts near the nipple and are referred to as subareolar abscesses; they are distinct conditions but their management is not dissimilar.

Although the management of patients with breast abscesses and lactational problems does not represent a large number of women seeking advice, nevertheless they are a source of considerable morbidity if improperly managed.

## Peripheral breast abscess (Fig. 7.1)

Peripheral non-puerperal breast abscesses are more common in pre-menopausal than in the postmenopausal women in a ratio of 3:1. They may be associated with other diseases such as diabetes or rheumatoid arthritis, steroid treatment, trauma to the breasts, or silicone or paraffin implants, but

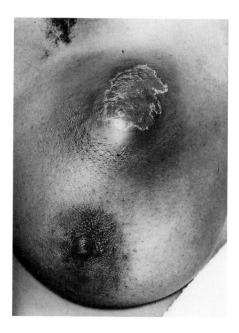

**Fig 7.1**  Peripheral abscess – a 3 × 2 cm fluctuant swelling can be seen in the upper outer quadrant of the breast. The surrounding area is erythematous with skin oedema and imminent necrosis over the most central part of the abscess.

they commonly present without any obvious predisposing factor. Their aetiology is unknown but may be associated with stasis of duct secretions in the smaller duct radicles. Bacteriological examination often demonstrates *Staphylococcus aureus* but more and more evidence is accumulating that anaerobic organisms – for example, *Bacteroides melaninogenicus*, *Bacteroides bivius*, and *Peptostreptococcus* spp. – are present as well suggesting a synergistic relationship.[1] The history is usually of 3 or 4 days duration, although on occasions this may extend up to several weeks before advice is sought. Characteristically the patient presents with a lump which is tender and may be associated with inflammatory changes in the skin with accompanying oedema of the breast. In contrast to puerperal breast abscess it is much less common to have any systemic evidence of malaise or fever.

*Management*

On first presentation patients should be examined carefully and an attempt made to obtain pus from the lesion, providing that it is not a well established abscess. Culture should be undertaken for aerobes and anaerobes and a suitable broad spectrum antibiotic mixture such as flucloxacillin and metronidazole or Augmentin should be started with early follow up in 24 or 48 hours. Undoubtedly if appropriate early treatment is started a substantial number of women will not go on to form overt abscesses.[2, 3] Should an abscess become established in spite of antibiotics then surgical treatment is indicated.

*Surgery*

Surgical treatment of an established peripheral abscess should be undertaken under a general anaesthetic, and an appropriately large skin incision made over the abscess cavity with careful digital examination carried out to ensure that all loculi of pus are broken down. Following this the abscess cavity should be actively curetted to remove the membranes separating the surrounding vascular breast from the abscess cavity. It is always worth excising a part of the wall for histology as occasionally carcinomas that have undergone necrosis can mimic the more common pyogenic abscess. The wound may then be closed by primary suture and the patient kept under observation either as an inpatient or an outpatient for 48 hours.[4] Excising the granulating cavity wall enables adequate therapeutic concentrations of antibiotics to penetrate all viable tissues surrounding the cavity; these should be administered orally for 5 to 7 days. Benson and Goodman[5] have shown that healing is quicker in primarily sutured wounds (21 days) than in those treated by the more classical method of incision and drainage (28 days). Unfortunately both methods of treatment still lead to a recurrence of abscesses of between 8 and 15%.[5, 6]

Despite the undoubted reduction in the number of patients presenting to hospital with peripheral breast abscesses, occasionally patients present with an obvious synergistic infection. In such instances the breast appears hard and indurated with associated skin erythema and axillary lymphadenopathy; it is often necessary to incise the breast to remove small pockets of pus. These patients, who may well have over half of their breast tissue involved in the inflammatory process, are best managed by leaving the wound open and using conventional Eusol and paraffin dressings. Management by excision and primary closure would lead to loss of a large amount of breast tissue, and suturing a wound in the presence of residual sepsis usually leads to wound breakdown and delayed healing. Dressings should be changed at least once daily until the cavity is clean, and then subsequent management can be with a Silastic foam dressing that is cleaned daily by the patient and supervised by the district nurse. Using this method healing of even large cavities will be completed in 6 to 10 weeks with a resulting linear scar, and a cosmetic result which is perfectly acceptable and often superior to a more conventional attempt at excision and closure of the wound.

Occasionally an antibioma will develop if there has been a delay in the onset of treatment or perhaps an inappropriate antibiotic has been prescribed. This disaster can be avoided by following the basic principle of treating an established abscess by surgery, and witholding antibiotics unless combined with surgical excision and primary drainage. The antibioma presents as a firm often hard swelling in the breast of a woman with a previous history and physical signs of an abscess. Treatment is most easily affected by careful surgical excision with primary closure using a suction drain; no antibiotic cover will be necessary if the antibioma is excised intact.

Traumatic fat necrosis may occasionally be mistaken for a peripheral breast abscess. The classical history follows a blunt injury with the development after 10 to 14 days of a hard mass with skin tethering and erythema.

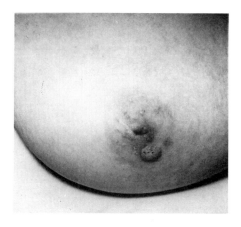

**Fig 7.2** Subareolar absecess – a small abscess can be seen on the inferior margin; this is associated with partial nipple inversion.

Traumatic fat necrosis usually affects the superficial subcutaneous fat rather than breast parenchyma proper, and the resulting inflammatory mass shows liquefaction of fat and infiltration of inflammatory cells – mostly lymphocytes and plasma cells.

## Subareolar breast abscesses

Subareolar breast abscesses present a different clinical problem. Patients are older but commonly premenopausal and non-puerperal, over half of them having some degree of anatomical nipple abnormality such as partial nipple inversion or nipple retraction. Fig. 7.2 shows a typical example of a patient with a subareolar abscess. The swelling can be seen in the lower part of the areola and it is accompanied by nipple inversion. Usually these patients present with intense subareolar pain often associated with a small palpable lesion. Often recurrent abscesses occur as can be seen in Fig. 7.3 where there are three circum areola incisions from previous episodes of infection; there is also a developing area of sepsis on the periphery of the areola at 1 o'clock.

*Aetiology*

The aetiology of subareolar breast inflammation is better understood than that of the peripheral lesion. Two processes have been implicated: abnormal squamous epithelial metaplasia[1] or mammary duct ectasia.[7] In the normal lactiferous duct there is an abrupt transition of squamous to columnar epithelium 1–2 mm beneath the surface of the nipple. Habif *et al*[8] noted that 17% of their patients with subareolar breast abscesses had squamous epithelium to an abnormal depth in the lactiferous duct. They noted extensive squamous replacement of the lining of one or more nipple ducts with obstruction by keratin plugs. This was followed by secondary ductal dilation caused by accumulation of ductal secretory material and cell debris. They noted that rupture of these ducts occurred with or without bacterial infection.

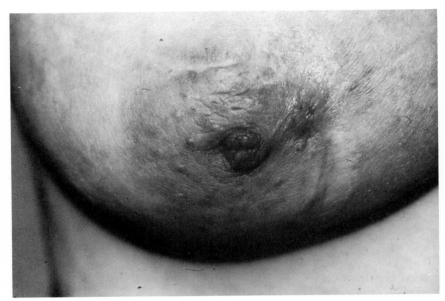

**Fig 7.3** Recurrent subareolar sepsis – surgical incisions from previously drained subareolar abscesses can be seen around the upper and medial parts of the areolar margin with a further subareolar abscess presenting within the previously incised area.

Mammary duct ectasia has been described by Haagensen[7] as an inflammatory disease of the major duct systems deep to the nipple and areola. Histologically there is periductal inflammation around the dilated ducts which contain cellular debris and lipid rich material; this inflammation leads eventually to fibrosis of the terminal ducts giving rise to shortening and eventual retraction of the nipple. Such ectasia is present in approximately 60% of postmenopausal women[9] but not all of these go on to develop periductal mastitis. It has been postulated by some authors[10] that these abnormalities in the ductal system may give rise to conditions favourable for bacteriological implantation, and they cite 3 cases of breast abscesses associated with nipple inversion which developed following a gynaecological examination, the cultures from the breast and the vagina both being *Bacteroides fragilis*, a commensal of the vagina.

Not all episodes of subareolar inflammation are bacteriological in origin, and in some studies a quarter of the patients have been noted to have duct ectasia with a chemical type of inflammatory reaction leading to a clinical manifestation of abscess or infection. This may, however, reflect difficulty in transporting and culturing anaerobic organisms. Bundret *et al*[11] found that by using appropriate transport media they could, in a high proportion of cases, culture both aerobic and anaerobic organisms from the ductal secretions of patients with duct ectasia and from all patients with periareolar sepsis.

*Treatment*

The confusion over surgical treatment of subareolar abscesses is in part a reflection of the diversity of opinion as to their aetiology. Those who favour abnormal squamous epithelial metaplasia suggest that surgical treatment should be by incision and drainage of pus followed by an excision of the abscess cavity and the communicating lactiferous sinus as a one stage operation.[12] Others, however, suggest that the drainage should be followed by a delayed excision of the fistulous tract,[13] as any communication can be more easily seen after the inflammatory process is quiescent. Many authors have reported clinical success following excision and saucerisation of mammary duct (mammillary) fistulas.[14]

For women presenting with early subareolar sepsis Rosenthal *et al*[3] have suggested needle aspiration with appropriate systemic antibiotic therapy as a first line of treatment. Using this method they have experienced a 10% abscess recurrence rate with no fistulae as a result of aspiration. This is in contrast to the experience of other authors who quote a recurrence rate following drainage of subareolar sepsis from around 40%[6, 12] to 75%.[15] Most recurrences occurred within the first year of treatment and most were in women who had a nipple abnormality, such as partial inversion or retraction.

It could be postulated that recurrence is a result of the failure of recognition and excision of the fistulous tract leading from the abscess cavity to the subareolar infection site, and the advice of incision and drainage followed by delayed exploration would hopefully reduce the incidence of recurrent infection. An example of a mammary duct fistula is shown in Fig. 7.4; the

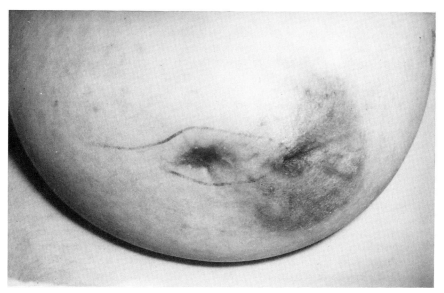

**Fig 7.4** Mammary duct fistula – nipple inversion associated with a long standing granulomatous fistulous tract at the areolar margin.

patient initially presented with a subareolar abscess which was treated by simple incision and several months later she presented with persistent subareolar sepsis and a mammary duct fistula. In this particular instance excision of the fistula track to the nipple including the adjacent lacteriferous duct resulted in eradication of the problem. Other authors[6] have suggested that all mammary duct fistulas show evidence of chronic inflammation, debris, and dilated ducts, satisfying the pathological definition of duct ectasia given by Azzopardi[16] and they will therefore need more extensive surgical treatment than simple ductal excision.

Infection of a sebaceous gland within the areola may give rise to an abscess which mimics the appearance of a subareolar lesion. In these cases one would expect that simple excision would result in permanent cure and it may be such cases as these that have lead some authors to advocate simple excision and closure as there would obviously be no communication with a lactiferous sinus and no risk of a mammary duct fistula.

*Acute Subareolar abscess* – The abscess cavity can be entered by incision at the periphery of the areola, pus then evacuated, and a sample retained for culture and sensitivity. The abscess cavity is then carefully explored with a probe in an attempt to identify any fistulous connection with a major lactiferous duct. Should this prove possible then excision of the major duct to its exit at the nipple and including the whole of the abscess cavity can be done as an *en bloc* dissection, and after careful haemostasis the cavity can be closed with interrupted fine sutures. Under appropriate antibiotic cover postoperative healing is straightforward.

*Mammary duct (mamillary) fistula* – Treatment is aimed at excising the infected granulomatous cavity in continuity with its mammary duct connection. Under general anaesthesia the mammary duct fistula is carefully probed until the communication with the nipple can be identified. Once this has been achieved with certainty then excision can proceed with an elliptical incision to include the skin over the mammary duct fistula with extension up on to the nipple to include the exit of the identified lactiferous sinus. After the skin incision is completed, subcutaneous dissection is deepened to include the whole of the abscess cavity together with a portion of breast distally to ensure that no major ductal system exists to enable further fistula formation. Careful inspection of the breast cavity will reveal any residual dilated ducts; if these are encountered further excision of breast parenchyma should proceed distally to reduce the risk of persistent inflammatory problems. This is an important technical point as it is possible for the major duct systems to become occluded by fibrosis with resultant dilation of peripheral ducts and subsequent inflammatory problems located more peripherally in the breast. After adequate haemostasis the wound can be closed by primary suture. As wound breakdown and subsequent delayed healing can result, many authors recommend that wounds be left open and allowed to heal by secondary intention. Providing that the wound can be kept clean and daily dressings applied using Eusol and paraffin (or, if appropriate, Silastic foam) then healing should be complete within 6 to 8 weeks.

*Recurrent subareolar infection*

In a proportion of patients there is recurrent infection at different sites and these are problems best managed by excision of the duct system as originally suggested by Patey and Thackray.[17]

The operation described by Hadfield[18] is carried out through an incision occupying about half the circumference of the areola; it is more convenient if the incision is placed over the site of maximum induration as this will lead to an easier dissection. After completion of the skin incision the nipple areola complex is dissected off the underlying breast tissue in a plane just deep to the subdermal veins. Once dissection has proceeded across the undersurface of the areola the nipple can be inverted with a fingertip and all remaining ductal tissue carefully dissected off the undersurface; if the nipple had previously been inverted a purse string suture of absorbable material can be used to maintain eversion during healing. The major ducts are excised *en bloc* in a cone of tissue the full diameter of the areola and extending 2–3 cm deep into the breast, ensuring that no dilated ducts remain. Haemostasis is achieved in the resulting cavity by diathermy or occasionally by directly placed sutures. Attempts can be made to close the cavity by 2 or 3 rows of purse string sutures starting deep in the wound, each subsequent purse string being more superficial. This, however, unfortunately often results in deformity of the breast and a better cosmetic result can usually be obtained by closing the original incision without any attempt to obliterate the cavity in the breast; haematoma formation is prevented by suction drains which are removed on the second or third postoperative day.

Occasional complications of surgery include partial loss of the areola as a result of ischaemia, but this can be avoided if the correct tissue plane is maintained during dissection. Many of the patients have an improved cosmetic result as the operation may result in permanent eversion of the nipple. In patients who have widespread mammary duct ectasia care needs to be taken to extend the incision far enough in the breast to remove all dilated systems. If this is not carried out adequately then recurrent abscess formation may necessitate further excision.

## Conclusions

The successful management of non-puerperal breast abscesses is dependent upon a thorough understanding of the underlying anatomical and pathological abnormality as well as on the recognition of the importance of mixed aerobic and anaerobic infection. Early use of an appropriate antibiotic should successfully resolve a large number of the lesions in patients presenting with subareolar infection. Of those that persist, subsequent management will depend upon isolating the underlying aetiological factors and carrying out appropriate surgery.

## Miscellaneous

Unusual breast abscesses may present as a result of diseases such as tuberculosis, actinomycosis, typhoid, or syphillis; all of these are extremely rare and likely to be diagnosed only after examination of the abscess cavity by histology and appropriate culture of the contained pus. Rarely a retromammary abscess may present as a complication of an empyema or tuberculous involvement of a costal cartilage or rib; drainage should follow basic surgical principles and in these instances a surgical approach through the inframammary fold has obvious advantages for dependent drainage.

Whilst there is usually little doubt about the diagnosis of infection in the breast one should be aware of the rare presentation of large inflammatory carcinomas of the breast with physical signs identical to those of an abscess; in cases where there may be doubt about the underlying diagnosis a Tru-cut biopsy may be necessary.

## Problems with lactation

### Non-puerperal lactation

Nipple discharge is not an uncommon complaint and one that is frequently referred for specialist opinion. The discharge is usually unilateral but may be bilateral and may consist of secretions from a single or multiple ducts. In most instances the colour is white or cream but varies from clear to dark – almost black – and is simply the result of normal ductal physiological secretion. Occasionally there may be a blood stained discharge which obviously has diagnostic implications for intraduct papillomas or carcinoma. Typically the patient complaining of non-puerperal lactation has a persistent profuse discharge of whitish fluid from several ducts on both nipples. This may be produced on only light pressure around the nipple but in some women is spontaneously produced in sufficient quantities to mark their underclothes constantly.

Prolactin, the stimulus for normal lactation, is controlled by hypothalamic inhibition, in the main by dopamine; many drugs which are dopamine antagonists can cause hyperprolactinaemia, which may or may not be associated with galactorrhoea. Occasionally patients who present with galactorrhoea have hyperprolactinaemia secondary to a prolactin secreting chromophobe adenoma (prolactinoma); in these patients amenorrhoea is a usual accompanying symptom (*see chapter 6*).

The commonest causes for non-puerperal lactation are either mechanical stimulation or oral contraception, although in the presence of amenorrhoea one should seriously consider the possible diagnosis of prolactinoma. In those rare instances where prolactinoma is the cause of galactorrhoea symptoms can be easily controlled by suppression of prolactin by using the drug bromocriptine.

If symptoms from a single duct are severe and persistent then a microdochectomy is a useful surgical procedure both to establish the cause (such as an intraduct papilloma) and to achieve symptomatic relief.

### Lactational problems during pregnancy

During the early weeks of pregnancy the breasts enlarge and become more vascular. Production of colostrum occurs from the sixteenth week of pregnancy onwards although this rarely appears at the nipple. The total volume increase in each breast is around 250 ml for most women. This results from ductal growth under the control of oestrogens, and acinar growth under the influence of progesterone and oestrogen; in addition human placental lactogen, prolactin, insulin, cortisol, and thyroxine all have an action on breast development during pregnancy. Rarely secondary breast development may occur along the nipple line in rudimentary breast tissue.

The principle hormonal stimulus for lactation – prolactin – is raised twentyfold during pregnancy, but its action is inhibited by high circulating oestrogens until after delivery. Following the rapid fall in circulating oestrogens, prolactin activates lactation which is maintained thereafter by suckling. Suckling also induces the secretion of oxytocin which activates the myoepithelial cells leading to 'let down' of milk. During the first few days of lactation colostrum alone is produced, but this should be actively encouraged by frequent application of the baby to the breast as once the colostrum has been expelled normal production of milk ensues.

Attempts to reduce the incidence of minor nipple trauma during feeding by the application of creams to the breast and nipple area during the later stage of pregnancy is widely recommended, but may not be very effective.

The simplest problem observed during breast feeding is soreness of the nipple due to trauma which can progress to cracking or fissuring. This can easily be treated by application of an aqueous cream without impeding breast feeding. Should nipple discomfort be a persistent problem then expression of the milk manually can be used until pain subsides sufficiently to allow normal suckling to recommence. Manual expression is carried out by massaging the breast from the periphery to the centre with ejection of milk being effected by pressure around the aerolar margin in a central direction deep into the breast.

Engorgement of either the whole breast or a segment may give rise to a local lump associated with considerable oedema and pain. This is often transient and can be satisfactorily treated by simple analgesics with manual expression until feeding can be painlessly recommenced. Occasionally in patients who have severe early engorgement of the breast, injection of oxytocin may help to initiating the milk 'let down' reflex. If engorgement persists and the mother wishes to stop breast feeding this can be assisted by firmly supporting the breast, avoiding nipple stimulation, and the use of a mild analgesic. Suppression of lactation is usually complete within 5 to 10 days when the breasts begin normal involution.

There is no longer a place for the use of stilboestrol in the prevention of lactation because of the increased risk of thromboembolic episodes, but bromocryptine can be used at a dose of 2.5 mg daily on the first postpartum day. Suppression of lactation can be achieved by bromcriptine 2.5 mg twice daily for 14 days, although this is not widely used because of its rather prominent and persistent side effects, the commonest of which are nausea and headaches.

## Galactocele

Normally after abrupt cessation of lactation the epithelial tissue in the breast rapidly involutes; this is not always in a uniform pattern and may lead to the development of a galactocele. The classical presentation would be of a discrete possibly cystic or firm lump in a woman who is lactating or has just finished lactation. Treatment should be by needle aspiration which will result in disappearance of the lump. Once aspirated it is unusual for a galactocele to reaccumulate and there is no need for this to affect the patient's wish to continue breast feeding. Surgical excision of a lump is never indicated as all can be successfully treated by simple aspiration and reassurance.

The galactocele consists of a collection of milk constituents secreted by hyperplastic lobular tissue which accumulate in breast ducts as shown by the presence of elastic fibres within the wall of the galactocele.[19]

## Acute puerperal mastitis

This condition, once epidemic in hospitals because of carriers of staphylococci, is now rather uncommon; there are, however, still sporadic endemic cases. The true incidence is difficult to ascertain but is probably as low as 1% of postpartum women. Most women present during the second and third weeks of lactation and, unless appropriate treatment is started within 24 hours, abscess development seems inevitable over the subsequent 7 to 10 days. There is no good evidence that either the baby or the mother suffers any ill effect from continued breast feeding and it may be that milk expression is beneficial in that it relieves pain and reduces the potential culture volume for bacteria. About 10% of women who experience mastitis in one pregnancy will have trouble in a subsequent pregnancy.

The patient typically presents in the second or third week of lactation with a painful lump in the breast associated with local oedema and often systemic upset and fever. Although cessation of breast feeding is not essential about half of the patients will spontaneously abandon breast feeding. There seems to be a definite reduction in the incidence of puerperal breast abscesses referred to hospital[1, 2, 20]; this may be due to improvement in perinatal care, and possibly a decreased incidence in the number of women engaging in breast feeding. There is no doubt, however, that early action in making a diagnosis and starting appropriate therapy will prevent development of an abscess in a substantial number of patients.

### Management

Most puerperal breast abscesses are due to *Staphylococcus aureus* or *Staphylococcus epidermidis* and over half are resistant to treatment with penicillin. An appropriate antibiotic such as flucloxacillin or Augmentin should be started immediately the condition is diagnosed. Administration of flucloxacillin should be half to one hour before food at a dose of 250 mg six hourly.

Augmentin has a wide bacteriocidal range and may be a more appropriate antibiotic for first line treatment; dosage is one tablet 8 hourly. The length of administration of oral antibiotics in the treatment of breast abscesses should be at least 5 days but should be continued longer if there is any doubt about complete resolution of symptoms. Should initial treatment prove ineffective and a true abscess develop then this should be treated by incision and drainage of the pus.

An adequate skin incision is made over the most fluctuant part of the lump, preferably following Langer's lines, or if appropriate at the margin of the areola. A specimen of the pus should be taken for culture and the abscess cavity carefully explored by digital exploration in order to break down all loculi. The abscess cavity should then be carefully curetted following which the wound may be closed either in primary fashion or incorporating a drain.

# References

1. Leach RD, Phillips I, Eykyn SJ, Corrie B. Anaerobic subareolar breast abscess *Lancet* 1979; **i**: 34–37.
2. Benson EA. Breast abscesses and breast cysts. *Practitioner* 1982; **226**: 1397–1401.
3. Rosenthal LJ, Greenfield DS, Lesnick GJ. Breast abscess. Management in subareolar and peripheral disease. *NY State J Med* 1981; **81**: 182–83.
4. Jones NAG, Wilson DH. The treatment of acute abscesses by primary suture under antibiotic cover. *Br J Surg* 1976; **63**: 499–501.
5. Benson EA, Goodman MA. Incision with primary suture in the treatment of acute puerperal breast abscess. *Br J Surg* 1970; **57**: 55–58.
6. Ekland DA, Zeigler MG. Abscess in the nonlactating breast. *Arch Surg* 1973; **107**: 398–401.
7. Haagensen CD. *Diseases of the Breast*. 2nd ed. Philadelphia, WB Saunders, 1971, 190–201.
8. Habif DV, Perzin KH, Lipton RL, Laites R. Subareolar abscess associated with squamous metaplasia of the lactiferous ducts. *Am J Surg* 1970; **119**: 523–26.
9. Tedeschi LG, Saeed A, Byrne JJ. Involutional mammary duct ectasia and periductal mastitis. *Am J Surg* 1963; **106**: 517–21.
10. Leach RD, Eykyn SJ, Phillips I. Vaginal manipulation and anaerobic breast abscesses. *Br Med J* 1981; **282**: 610–11.
11. Bundred NJ, Dixon JMJ, Lumsden AB, *et al*. Are the lesions of duct ectasia sterile? *Br J Surg* 1985; **72**: 844–45.
12. Watt-Boolsen S, Rasmussen NR, Blichert-Toft M. Primary periareolar abscess in the nonlactating breast: risk of recurrence. *Am J Surg* 1987; **153**: 571–3.
13. Maier WP, Berger A, Derrick BM. Periareolar abscess in the non lactating breast. *Am J Surg* 1982; **144**: 359–61.
14. Lambert ME, Betts CD, Sellwood RA. Mammary fistulae. *Br J Surg* 1986; **73**: 367–68.
15. Scholefield JH, duncan JL, Rogers K. Review of a hospital experience of breast abscesses. *Br J Surg* 1987; **76**: 469–70.
16. Azzopardi JC. *Problems in Breast Pathology*. Eastbourne, WB Saunders & Co, 1979, 72–75.
17. Patey DH, Thackray AC. Pathology and treatment of mammary duct ectasia. *Lancet* 1958; **ii**: 871–73.

18. Hadfield J. Excision of the major system for benign disease of the breast. *Br J Surg* 1960; **48**: 472–77.
19. Ironside JW, Guthrie W. The galactocoele: a light and electronmicroscopic study. *Histopathology* 1985; **9**: 457–67.
20. Bates T, Down RHL, Tant DR, Fiddian RV. The current treatment of breast abscesses in hospital and in general practice. *Practitioner* 1973; **211**: 541–47.

# 8

# Benign neoplastic disease–pathological considerations for high risk

DL PAGE

Assessment of risk for later carcinoma development is an impelling interest of physicians who treat breast disease. These putative determinants have changed during this century, and will continue to do so. For example, in the first half of this century it was believed that mammary cysts were closely related to carcinoma and until recently it was widely believed that cysts of palpable size were markers of increased breast cancer risk. A discussion of cysts also allows for the recognition that other histologic changes are frequently associated with cysts and were noted by Foote and Stewart[1] in the 1940s as part of the complex termed 'fibrocystic disease'. While it is certainly true that these various changes (hyperplasia, fibrosis, cysts, adenosis, and apocrine change) tend to occur together, it is their separate evaluation in defined groups of women which allow for the identification of increased cancer risk. Cyst formation as a single determinant is not an indicator of increased risk in a single ethnic group.[2] Interestingly, cysts are more common in ethnic groups with higher risk of breast cancer than they are in those of lower risk (Hispanic and Indian women of New Mexico) as demonstrated by Bartow et al.[3] The separate analysis of each reliably indentifiable histological feature should be the hallmark of risk assessment, and this presentation is dedicated to this approach.

Risk assessment using histological markers should be understood for both biological and practical purposes to have interactions with other risk indicators. These non-anatomical indicators of greatest interest are mammographic pattern, late age at first birth, and family history of breast cancer. These interactions have been best studied with regard to family history[2] and age at first birth.[4] Considering the relative ease with which mammographic information may be obtained as compared to a breast biopsy specimen, this will be a useful approach. Recently a correlation between nodular densities on mammography and histological epithelial hyperplasia has been reported.[5] The relationship of dense mammographic patterns to increased breast cancer risk is supported by a careful review of published reports.[6] The magnitude and sub groups relevant to this increased risk, however, have not as yet been clarified by prospective studies.

## Background

The data supporting the guidelines presented here derive primarily from a large prospective study performed in Nashville, Tennessee. Thus the histology was evaluated as it was present at the time follow up began – that is, at the time of initial surgical biopsy. A total of 10 542 breast biopsy specimens originally diagnosed as benign were histologically reviewed. These had been performed at the three major hospitals of this city between 1950 and 1968.[2] All women with proliferative changes were followed for the development of invasive breast carcinoma, as were a similar number of women without proliferative changes. The 3303 women who were followed an average of 17 years after benign breast biopsy represented a follow up success rate of 84.4%. Similar studies are few, but have supported the positive relationship between epithelial hyperplasia and increased breast cancer risk.[7–9]

The categories indicating magnitude of risk (Table 8.1) are derived from a consensus statement which followed the publication of the Nashville studies.[10] The phrases are meant to indicate that the lesions involved are histological and the paired risk statements emphasise the clinical implications by stating the magnitude of risk for later development of invasive carcinoma. Note that these statements are made with the assumption that carcinoma *in situ* is a high risk lesion. Note also that carcinoma *in situ* in this setting is understood to indicate carcinoma *in situ* of lobular type and microscopic examples of ductal carcinoma *in situ*.

The historical inspiration and background for these studies of risk assessment extend back to the early part of this century and include most prominently the names of Joseph Colt Bloodgood, R Muir, Arthur Purdy Stout, James Ewing, Edith Dawson, Fred Stewart, and Frank Foote. The criteria developed in the careful studies of Wellings *et al*[11] and Jensen *et al*[12] were taken into account as noted below in setting histological criteria. These workers attempted to describe the total pathological content of the human breast using primarily slices through the complete breast and viewing with a dissecting microscope. A scheme of quantitating histological and cytologic patterns with placement in a range of histological change was also used by Black and Chabon[13] in a similar fashion.

## No risk lesions

Within this category are found many changes which characterise the majority of benign breast biopsy specimens and include cysts of any size, mild hyperplasia of usual type, and apocrine change. It is likely that radial scars without the coexistence of significant epithelial hyperplasia should also be in this group, although formal prospective analysis of those lesions is not yet forthcoming except in studies of limited scope. In the consensus statement of the College of American Pathologists,[10] sclerosing adenosis was in this no risk category despite its inclusion in the group of slightly increased risk lesions, designated proliferative disease without atypia, by Dupont and Page.[2] This was deemed appropriate because of the lack of prior support for sclerosing adenosis as an indicator of increased risk. Subsequent specific analysis of sclerosing adenosis within this large study from Nashville, however,[14] has indicated that sclerosing adenosis does indicate a risk in this low range which is not accounted for by the co-occurrence of this change with other elements of proliferative disease without atypia. It is still important for this finding to be supported by other studies, and McDivitt *et al*[15] provide support for the inclusion of sclerosing adenosis in the slightly increased risk group.

Mild epithelial hyperplasia of usual type is extremely common in breast biopsy specimens and is understood to indicate the increase in numbers of cells above the basement membrane area to a thickness of three or four, with the normal cell thickness understood to be two. These mild changes are also understood to lack features noted for moderate and florid hyperplasia of usual type discussed below.

Lesions in the no risk category may be viewed as defined by exclusion – that is, risk indicator lesions are absent. Seventy per cent of breast biopsy specimens were included in this group. There is actually some indication that women having this group of histological alterations are at slightly decreased risk compared with the general population as their overall risk, controlled for age and length of follow up, was 10% less than that of the general population. Although this decrease is not statistically or clinically significant, it adds credibility to the finding that these women undergoing biopsy are not at increased risk of subsequent carcinoma development.

## Slightly increased risk

The magnitude of increase of risk in this group is in the range of 1.5 to 2 times that of the general population controlled for age and time at risk. This recording of the increase of risk as a range is chosen in order to indicate that the indication is not specific but rather probabilistic. It is also true that if different comparison populations are used for these lesions then the risk varies within this range. Another way to relay this information is to say that risk is increased, but not reliably as much as doubled. A doubling of risk should be roughly understood to be of similar magnitude to that associated with a positive family history of breast cancer.

The major histological patterns found within this category are the usual or common types of epithelial hyperplasia. These changes are most frequent in the perimenopausal years and are often recognized by such terms as 'papillomatosis' and 'epitheliosis'. The diagnostic patterns are recognised by greater quantitative changes than mild hyperplasia, with cells crossing and distending spaces in which they reside. Atypical features noted below are absent. There is a characteristic mild variation in cytologic features and cell placement (Fig. 8.1). Our studies have used the terms moderate and florid hyperplasia without atypia, or proliferative disease without atypia, in order

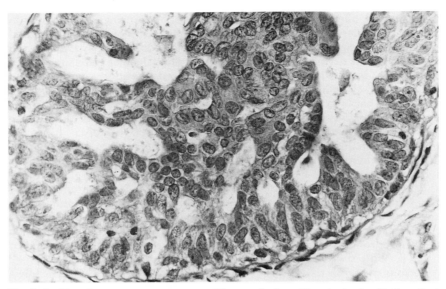

**Fig 8.1**  Usual or common pattern of hyperplasia without atypia. Notice that the cells form a pattern of nuclei which appear to swirl about (streaming). Also, nuclei vary considerably in shape, with round and oval nuclei readily apparent. the intercellular spaces are also irregular and frequently slit like. Thus despite the evident increased cellularity with mild nuclear pattern variation, there are no features of atypia.

to emphasise that some disorder as implied by the term 'disease' is present, specifically the indication of a slight increase in risk. The term 'without atypia' is added in order to specify in the diagnostic statement that those histological alterations associated with somewhat greater increase of risk are absent. Note that well developed, microscopic examples of sclerosing adenosis probably belong in this group as noted above. Papillomas of any type are also included here, although further study of their stratification by pattern and extent is warranted.

## Moderately increased risk

This term was chosen by a consensus conference[10] in order to place these lesions in perspective between those noted above and microscopic examples of *in situ* carcinoma. The relative risk for subsequent invasive carcinoma of the atypical hyperplasias within this group is four to five times that of the general population. This is approximately half the risk experienced by women with microscopic carcinoma *in situ* (see below).

The recognition that a woman has a risk relative to the general population of an approximate magnitude of four times demands clarification as it is easily misunderstood. These relative risk figures compare two groups for purposes of statistical evaluation, and are not readily transferred directly to clinical practice. This relative risk figure derived from our studies[16] is bound by the experience of the groups studied and is thus confined to the follow up period of approximately 15 years. It is also somewhat confined to the group of women who are most frequently biopsied in usual clinical practice – that is, those women about the age of 50. Few women of the ages less than 30 and more than 60 were present in our studies, and these risk figures must be understood to be less certain for women in these age groups.

The atypical hyperplastic lesions which comprise this risk group are recognised histologically by their close resemblance to lesions long recognised as carcinoma *in situ*. They are named by their analogy to lobular carcinoma *in situ* and ductal carcinoma *in situ*, respectively, and are histologically more resembling of their analogous carcinoma *in situ* lesions than the usual hyperplastic lesions. The atypical hyperplasias, as defined in this manner, may be viewed as having the same features as the carcinoma *in situ* lesions, but in less than fully developed form. Histological rules for separating the atypical hyperplastic lesions from carcinoma *in situ* lesions are not the same as those which separate the atypical hyperplastic lesions from hyperplasia without atypia, as the histological categories are not a continuum of alteration. Rather than being a continuum or range of change, these histological definitions were made in order to recognise natural groupings of lesions in the complex array of histological mammary alterations. The approach used was more that of the mammalogist naturalist seeking to identify separate species or sub species, or both, within a group of similar animals, from their anatomical characteristics.

As a result of this approach, the rules of histopathological definition may be viewed as having their complexity as a natural result of the complexity of patterns found in breast biopsy specimens. The separation of atypical lobular hyperplasia from lobular carcinoma *in situ* is based upon an arbitrary rule which we found most conducive to reproducibility in diagnosis. The categories produced by this separation were then tested in a prospective, epidemiological setting and found to indicate different levels of risk (Table 8.1). Lobular carcinoma *in situ* is recognised where there is a well developed example of filling, distention, and distortion of over half the acini of a lobular unit by a uniform population of characteristic cells. This follows the approach of the original discription.[17] Atypical lobular hyperplasia is recognised (Figs. 8.2 and 8.3) when more than half the acini are not completely distended, or filled by the uniform population of characteristic cells or both.[18] Further stratification of risk is attained by recognising the phenomenon of involvement by ducts of these uniform, round cells. This phenomenon has been long recognised as pagetoid spread into ducts.[17] When the lobular units involved only attain the features of atypical lobular hyperplasia, this ductal involvement has been termed ductal involvement by cells of atypical lobular hyperplasia.[19] It is clear from Table 8.2 that ductal involvement in cases otherwise qualifying as atypical lobular hyperplasia produces a subsequently increased risk of breast carcinoma close to or within the range recognised by lobular carcinoma *in situ*.

The last category in Table 8.2, minimal features of atypical lobular

**Table 8.1**   Relative risk* for invasive breast carcinoma based on histological examination of breast tissue without carcinoma[2 10]

---

- No increased risk (non-proliferative disease):
  Adenosis, sclerosing or florid†
  Duct estasia
  Mild epithelial hyperplasia of usual type.‡
- Slightly increased risk (1.5–2 times): (epithelial proliferative disease without atypia)
  Hyperplasia of usual type, moderate or florid
- Moderately increased risk (4–5 times): (atypical hyperplasia)¶
  Atypical ductal hyperplasia
  Atypical lobular hyperplasia
- High risk (8–10 times): (carcinoma *in situ*)§
  Lobular carcinoma *in situ*
  Non-comedo ductal carcinoma *in situ*

---

* Women in each category are compared to women matched for age who have had no breast biopsy with regard to risk of invasive breast cancer in the ensuring 10–20 years. † This lesion rests in the 'no elevation of risk' category despite the presentation by Dupont and Page[2] of sclerosing adenosis in the slightly increased risk category. Sclerosing adenosis had not been previously found to be associated with increased risk; McDivitt *et al*,[15] however also support a slight increase in cancer risk. ‡ These lesions are hyperplastic as they have ③ or ④ cells above a basement membrane, rather than the normal complement of 2. They also have little tendency to cross over spaces or distend spaces, while the moderate and florid hyperplasias often have ⑤ or more cells above the basement membrane and tend to cross and distend spaces. These latter, slightly increased risk lesions, are commonly recognised as 'papillomatosis', or 'epitheliosis' without atypia. ¶ The atypical hyperplastic lesions differ somewhat in age incidence and interval to appearance of later cancer,[16] but are associated with the same magnitude of increased risk. § Strict criteria for these lesions are used. Note that only smaller examples of non-comedoductal carcinoma have been assessed as risk indicators after biopsy only.

**Table 8.2**   Stratification of subsequent invasive breast cancer risk relative to variants of lobular neoplasia

|  | Relative risk of invasive carcinoma compared with general population of comparable age and length of time at risk |
|---|---|
| Lobular carcinoma *in situ* | 7–9 |
| Atypical lobular hyperplasia with ductal involvement[19] | 7 |
| Atypical lobular hyperplasia, no ductal involvement[19] | 3 |
| Suggestive changes with increase in cell number[19] | 1.7 |

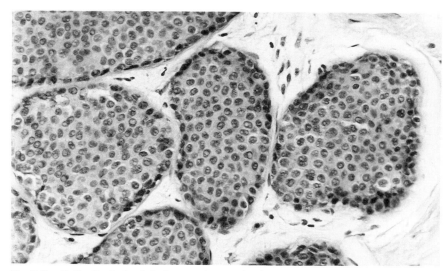

**Fig 8.2**   Full criteria for lobular carcinoma *in situ* are apparent in these few acini with filling and distension of each individual acinus by a uniform cell population.

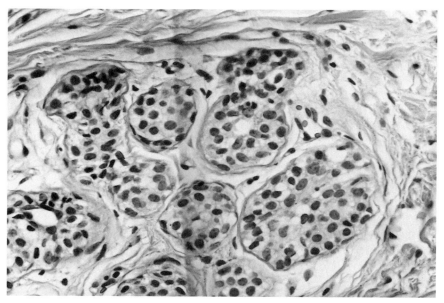

**Fig 8.3**   Atypical lobular hyperplasia is present with little distention of each of the acini within this lobular unit as well as residual intercellular lumina in several spaces.

hyperplasia, was recognised in our cohort study[19] in order to set the least confines of definition for this range of histological lesions. It is recognised when a lobular unit has the general appearance of atypical lobular hyperplasia, but increased number of cells cannot be reliably identified within acini. This end point of recognition of atypical lobular hyperplasia is present when it is not possible readily to identify more than four cells when counting nuclei from one basement membrane to the oppoite basement membrane within an acinus. In other words, the normal cell population of two cells above the basement membrane would produce the total counting of four cells when counting the full complement of cells across the diameter of an acinus. Mimicry of atypical lobular hyperplasia is often produced by poorly fixed specimens, and has been recognised in the past as mimicking lobular carcinoma *in situ*.[20]

Atypical ductal hyperplasia is less well established as a risk indicator than atypical lobular hyperplasia. The reason for this is simply that its demonstration of magnitude of risk rests upon a single study.[2, 14] Our first study, based on only 1000 cases,[21] demonstrated precisely the same increase in breast cancer risk for atypical lobular hyperplasia as was found in the later studies noted above. In that earlier study the category of atypical ductal hyperplasia was intermeshed with examples of florid hyperplasia and did not demonstrate a greater increase in risk than double. The confines of definition of atypical ductal hyperplasia are also less definite than those of the lobular series, although most cases may be reliably recognised. The diagnosis of atypical hyperplasia of ductal type must be recognised using the standard features which define ductal carcinoma *in situ*. Those features are noted in Table 8.3. Note that most commonly cases of atypical ductal hyperplasia demonstrate well developed features of ductal carcinoma *in situ*. There is a remaining cell population within the involved spaces, however, which appears normal in that it rests above a basement membrane and frequently above a layer of recognisable myoepithelial cells, demonstrates a polarity and orientation toward the lumen, and, most importantly, has no nuclear pattern similarity to the cells of the atypical cell population (Fig. 8.4).

Each type of atypical hyperplasia was found in follow up to indicate an increased risk of breast cancer in the range of four to five times that of the

**Table 8.3**  Histological criteria for cribriform and micropapillary carcinoma in situ

- Uniform population of cells throughout entire space bounded by basement membrane
- 'Punched out', neatly rounded, geometric spaces – or bulbous, well defined, papillary fronds.
- Round, hyperchromatic, monotonous, randomly placed nuclei
- Helpful: presence in many spaces (at least ②)

Modified from Page D L. Cancer risk assessment in benign breast biopsies. *Hum Pathol* 1986; **17**:871–74.

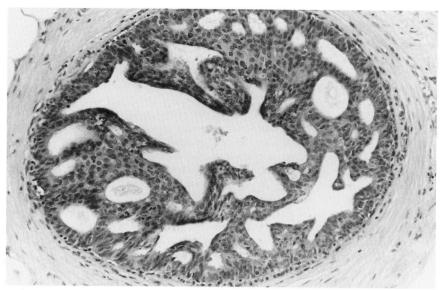

**Fig 8.4** Atypical ductal hyperplasia with a pattern of rigidity of arches, but without regularly round and sharply demarcated edges. Also, the population of cells lining the wall of the space are different, evenly polarised, and have much more cytoplasm, although not well appreciated at the lower power.

general population. There was such a strong interaction with family history in this study that it is relevant to consider women with atypical hyperplasia who have a positive family history of breast cancer separately from those who do not. The absolute risk of breast cancer development in women with atypical hyperplasia without a family history in 10 years was 8%, whereas those with a positive family history experienced a risk of about 25% at 15 years. This strong interaction with family history has not been verified in a later study with a different study design, although the atypical hyperplastic lesions did recognise an increase in risk of similar magnitude.[15] The risk for subsequent breast carcinoma development is equally distributed between either breast for both lesions of atypical lobular and atypical ductal hyperplasia.

## Lesions of increased risk

Histological lesions qualifying for this category are microscopic examples of ductal carcinoma *in situ* and lobular carcinoma *in situ*. Note that mass lesions produced by ductal carcinoma *in situ*, particularly comedoductal carcinoma *in situ*, are excepted from this category of high risk lesions.

Lobular carcinoma *in situ* is the classic example of a greatly increased risk lesion identifying a high risk of subsequent carcinoma development in either breast. The predictive utility of lobular carcinoma *in situ* is recorded in several studies, and recognises an increased risk in the range of 7 to 9 times that of the general population. No interaction to increase the magnitude of risk further has been recognised, even for the concurrence of a positive family history of breast cancer.[22, 23] Ductal involvement (pagetoid spread) in the presence of atypical lobular hyperplasia indicates an increase in risk approaching the magnitude of lobular carcinoma *in situ*.[19, 24]

Our understanding of the natural history of microscopic examples of ductal carcinoma *in situ* comes largely from two studies published in 1978 and 1982.[25, 26] Each of these studies reviewed a large number of breast biopsy specimens previously recognised as benign and identified a total of almost 60 cases of microscopic and non-comedoductal carcinoma *in situ*. Follow up of these women demonstrated an absolute risk of breast cancer development between 25 and 30% in 15 years. The relative risk of this experience was about 10 times that of the general population. Importantly, both studies were in total agreement that subsequent invasive carcinoma occurred in the same area of the breast as the originally identified carcinoma *in situ* lesions. This strongly indicates that such lesions are predominantly monofocal as tested by the biology of long term follow up.

These studies of carcinoma *in situ* have demonstrated the great difference between the ductal and lobular categories with regard to their indications for clinical management. It seems likely that relatively small and non-comedoductal examples of ductal carcinoma *in situ* may be cured by local excision. Only further experience will prove where in the range of size and histology this conservative approach might be most appropriate. There is a mounting experience with conservative treatment of ductal carcinoma *in situ*, however, which seems quite satisfactory for the microscopic lesions.

Lobular carcinoma *in situ* must be considered as an indicator of risk anywhere within both breasts. The experience of Haagensen *et al*[23] demonstrated that women who were closely followed after the demonstration of high risk lesions of lobular type were consistently alive and well following treatment by mastectomy of their later developing invasive breast cancers. This observation support the conserving clinical pasture of close follow up with the addition of mammography, which was not available to Haagensen *et al*, in the early detection of curable breast carcinomas in this setting. Thus many now apply close surveillance by mammography to women with lobular carcinoma *in situ*, although extirpative surgery is also used.

## Conclusions

Risk assessment of breast cancer development is an endeavour unfamiliar to most physicians. Our familiarity with risk assessment and its ease of use in a clinical setting will grow in the ensuing years. Of greatest importance to this growth will be the garnering of more specific information about determinants of risk and their interaction with screening and therapeutic modalities. Although trite, it is still true that more questions are raised than have been answered. We are not a full professional generation removed from a time when the question of malignancy in the breast was absolute, yes or no.

Now special types of breast cancer are recognised as being of little threat to life, and some benign lesions have an increased risk of cancer.

Of greatest practical importance currently is the fact that upwards of 70% of women undergoing biopsy of a benign breast lesion are not at increased risk of breast cancer development. This is to be understood against the background of prior wisdom that all such women were at 2–3 times the risk of the general population.

At the present, women with slightly increased risk might be encouraged to follow a regular (yearly) programme of mammographic surveillance, while women with lesions associated with moderately increased risk should follow such a programme without fail. Atypical hyperplasia is rare, occurring in only 4% of breast biopsy specimens prior to the mammographic era, although this incidence is currently higher with mammographically directed biopsy.[27] Other considerations such as mammographic density, family history, and high anxiety will impinge on the decisions made. In most of these patients, however, extirpative surgery is probably not a practical consideration.

# References

1. Foote FW, Stewart FW. Comparative studies of cancerous versus noncancerous breasts. *Ann Surg* 1945; **121**: 6–222.
2. Dupont WD, Page DL. Risk factors for breast cancer in women with proliferative breast disease. *N Engl J Med* 1985; **312**: 146–51.
3. Bartow SA, Pathak DR, Black WC, *et al.* Prevalence of benign, atypical, and malignant breast lesions in populations at different risk for breast cancer. *Cancer* 1987; **60**: 2751–60.
4. Dupont WD, Page DL. Breast cancer risk associated with proliferative disease, age at first birth, and a family history of breast cancer. *Am J Epidemiol* 1987; **125**: 769–79.
5. Bright RA, Morrison AS, Brisson J, *et al.* Relationship between mammographic and histologic features of breast tissue in women with benign biopsies. *Cancer* 1988; **61**: 266–71.
6. Boyd NF, O'Sullivan B, Fishell E, *et al.* Mammographic patterns and breast cancer risk: methodic standards and contradictory results. *JNCI* 1984; **72**: 1253–59.
7. Black MD, Barclay THC, Cutler SJ, *et al.* Association of atypical characteristics of benign breast lesions with subsequent risk of breast cancer. *Cancer* 1972; **29**: 338–43.
8. Kodlin D, Winger EE, Morgenstern NL, Chen U. Chronic mastopathy and breast cancer: a follow-up study. *Cancer* 1977; **39**: 2603–07.
9. Hutchinson WB, Thomas DB, Hamlin WB, *et al.* Risk of breast cancer in women with benign breast disease. *JNCI* 1980; **65**: 13–20.
10. Hutter RVP, and others. Consensus meeting. Is 'fibrocystic disease' of the breast precancerous? *Arch Pathol Lab Med* 1986; **110**: 171–73.
11. Wellings SR, Jensen HM, Marcum RG. An atlas of subgross pathology of the human breast with special reference to possible precancerous lesions. *JNCI* 1975; **55**: 231–73.
12. Jensen HM, Rice JR, Wellings SR. Preneoplastic lesions in the human breast. *Science* 1976; **191**: 295–97.

13. Black MM, Chabon AB. *In situ* carcinoma of the breast. *Pathol Annu* 1969; **4**: 185–210.
14. Jensen RA, Page DL, Dupont WD, Rogers LW. Invasive breast cancer (IBC) risk in women with sclerosing adenosis (SA). *Lab Invest* 1988; **56**: 43A.
15. McDivitt RW, Rubin GL, Stevens JA, *et al.* Benign breast disease histology and the risk of breast cancer: *Lab Invest* 1988; **58**: 62A.
16. Page DL, Dupont WD, Rogers LW, Rados MS. Atypical hyperplastic lesions of the female breast. *Cancer* 1985; **55**: 2698–708.
17. Foote FW, Stewart FW. Lobular carcinoma *in situ*. *Am J Pathol* 1941; **17**: 491–95.
18. Page DL, Anderson TJ. *Diagnostic Histopathology of the Breast.* Edinburgh, Churchill Livingstone, 1987.
19. Page DL, Dupont WD, Rogers LW. Ductal involvement by cells of atypical lobular hyperplasia in the breast: a long-term follow-up study of cancer risk. *Hum Pathol* 1988; **19**: 201–07.
20. McDivitt RW, Stewart FW, Berg JW. 1968 Tumors of the breast. In: *Atlas of Tumor Pathology, second series, fascicle 2.* Washington, Armed Forces Institute of Pathology, pp 72–77.
21. Page DL, Vander Zwaag R, Rogers LW, *et al.* Relation between component parts of the fibrocystic disease complex and breast cancer. *JNCI* 1978; **61**: 1055–63.
22. Rosen PP, Lieberman PH, Braun DW Jr, *et al.* Lobular carcinoma *in situ* of the breast: detailed analysis of 99 patients with average follow-up of 24 years. *Am J Surg Pathol* 1978; **2**: 225–51.
23. Haagensen CD, Lane N, Lattes R, Bodian C. Lobular neoplsia (so called lobular carcinoma *in situ*) of the breast. *Cancer* 1978; **42**: 737–69.
24. Page DL, Kidd TE, Dupont WD, Rogers LW. Lobular neoplasia of the breast has varying magnitudes of risk for subsequent invasive carcinoma. *Lab Invest* 1988; **58**: 69A.
25. Betsill WL Jr, Rosen PP, Lieberman PH, Robbins GF. Intraductal carcinoma. Long-term follow-up after treatment by biopsy alone. *JAMA* 1978; **239**: 1863–67.
26. Page DL, Dupont WD, Rogers LW, Landenberger M. Intraductal carcinoma of the breast: follow-up after biopsy only. *Cancer* 1982; **39**: 751–58.
27. Rubin E, Alexander RW, Visscher DW, *et al.* Proliferative disease and atypia in biopsies performed for mammographically detected nopalpable lesions. *Cancer,* 1988; **61**: 2077–2080

# 9

# Risk factors for benign breast disease

IS FENTIMAN

## Introduction

There is a large body of information about risk factors for breast cancer. Not surprisingly, the same epidemiological techniques have also been applied to the study of benign breast disease. Such investigations may be seriously flawed, however, if 'benign breast disease' is regarded as a well circumscribed and characterised disease entity. Benign breast disease may be defined as any non-malignant condition causing signs or symptoms relating to the breast, and it therefore encompasses a range of diseases and non-diseases. These may be more or less characterised clinically or pathologically and may have totally different relationships to subsequent risk of mammary malignancy.

Patients with breast cancer will, almost without exception, have had a biopsy for histological confirmation of the diagnosis because they developed either a breast mass or other symptoms or signs requiring treatment. Thus most of these cases will at least be characterised histologically. In contrast, the decision to carry out a biopsy for what is eventually diagnosed as a benign condition will depend upon a variety of factors, some of which will be non-biological. Thus surgical intervention may depend upon the ease of palpating the lump (as a result of subcutaneous fat distribution), access to surgical assessment, accidents of geography, ability to pay for treatment, and the patient's prior history and familial predisposition to malignancy.

Even when a biopsy has been performed the histological report may use terms that have different meanings for pathologist and surgeon, some of which may be circumlocutions for normality. There is a large group of women described as having benign breast disease, without being subjected to biopsy. Many of these have cyclical or non-cyclical mastalgia with or without nodularity. Thus the label 'benign breast disease' is an inappropriate conjunction of patients with lumps, lumpiness, pain, or nipple discharge and succeeds in producing a great deal of confusion. This is of particular concern because a few patients with histologically defined benign lesions are at increased risk of subsequent breast cancer. Most patients with surgically or medically treated benign breast problems do not carry any increased risk. This review will examine risk factors for defined groups of patients with benign problems. The problems will include fibroadenoma, fibrocystic disease, and mastalgia. The risk factors being considered will comprise age, weight, family history, contraceptive history and reproductive history, together with smoking and caffeine consumption. In addition the relationship between various benign lesions and subsequent cancer risk will be analysed.

## Fibroadenoma

These common lesions develop from lobules during pubertal growth or sometimes in response to lactation. Although histologically divisible into the pericanalicular type (with branched tubules within loose stroma) and intracanalicular type (with epithelial cyst formation, collapse and invagination of cyst walls), the two types may coexist. None of the epidemiological studies so far carried out have considered separately the two sub types. Most of these lesions become clinically apparent between the ages of 15 and 25. Many women, however, have silent fibroadenomas which, because of their deep location within dense breast tissue, will be undetected clinically. Standard surgical teaching has been that all palpable, discrete breast lumps should be removed, but this is being increasingly questioned. Thus many surgeons confronted with a woman aged less than 25 with a clinically suspected fibroadenoma will confirm this cytologically, and leave the lump unbiopsied. Nevertheless, despite the surgeon being satisfied about the diagnosis many patients will still be anxious and at present most women prefer to have the lump removed and its nature confirmed histologically.[1]

### Risk factors for fibroadenoma

*Age*

The age incidence figures from four case control series which present comparable data have been combined and are shown in Fig. 9.1.[2-5] This indicates that the peak incidence occurs between the ages of 15 and 24 and also the inverse relationship between age and incidence. There is a slight increase in detection among women aged over 65, which is probably a result of the fatty replacement of breast tissue which unmasks the fibroadenoma and, despite the absence of signs of malignancy, the lesion will almost always be excised in a woman in this age group. Many fibroadenomas are undetected clinically and this has been confirmed in the study of Frantz *et al* who examined parallel gross sections of breast tissue from a sequential series of 225 autopsies of females dying from non-breast-related conditions.[6] The peak incidence was in those aged less than 19 but fibroadenomas were found in almost all age groups up to 89 years (Fig. 9.2). These findings are also supported by mammographic studies on asymptomatic screened women in

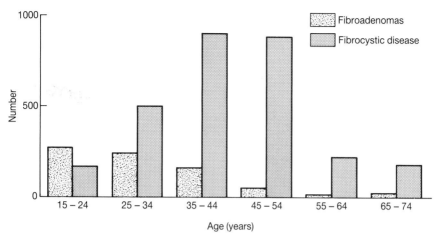

**Fig 9.1** Comparison of age distribution of patients with fibroadenomas and fibrocystic disease.

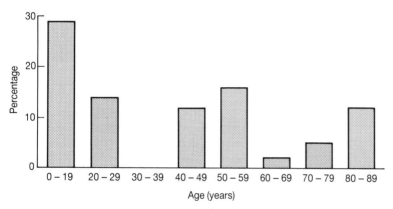

**Fig 9.2** Age distribution in autopsy series[6].

which calcified or non-calcified fibroadenomas are being found in patients of all ages.[7]

*Weight*

It has been consistently reported that there is an inverse relationship between body weight and incidence of fibroadenomas. Thus when weight is directly measured, and taking the relative risk as unity for women weighing less than 55 kg, this falls to a relative risk of 0.4 for women over 65 kg.[8] Similarly, indirect measurement by Quetelet's index shows that a relative risk of one for those women with an index less than 21 falls to 0.2 for those fat women whose index is greater than 25.[3] It is unlikely that there is any direct aetiological relationship between leanness and fibroadenomas. A much more likely explanation is the ease of detection of breast lumps in thin individuals.

## Reproductive features

The effects of age at menarche, nulliparity, and age at first pregnancy as risk factors for fibroadenoma are given in Table 9.1, in which the results from 9 case control studies which specifically gave data on patients with biopsy proven fibroadenomas are summarised.[2, 3, 5, 8-13] Age at menarche was not shown to be a risk factor in most of the studies, although Cole reported a relative incidence of 1.7 for women who started menstruation after the age of 12.[3] In contrast, Parazzini *et al* found a relative risk of 1.5 for those who menstruated before the age of 14.[13]

Most case control studies have shown an increasing risk for nulliparous women. Rather than suggesting that pregnancy protects against fibroadenoma development, however, a more likely explanation is that more women develop fibroadenomas at an age before they will have become pregnant, thereby artificially creating a moderate increase in relative risk for nulliparity. When age is controlled for, the effect of nulliparity is lost.[3] Age at first pregnancy, which is an important risk factor for breast carcinoma, has not been shown to have any effect on risk of development of fibroadenomas.

## Family history of breast cancer

Kelsey *et al*[9] reported that a family history of breast cancer had no effect on risk of fibroadenomas. Nomura *et al*[10] found that patients with fibroadenomas reported a family history more frequently than controls, although this could have been a chance finding. Ravnihar[11] also observed a slight but non-significant increase in family history in patients with fibroadenomas but postulated that this was due to heightened breast awareness. Certainly, no clear cut association has emerged between family history of breast cancer and risk of fibroadenoma.

## Socioeconomic factors

There have been seven case control studies which examined indices of wealth, social class and education and the results of these are given in Table 9.2.[3, 4, 8, 10-13] The findings are remarkably consistent. Women from social class 1 have an increased incidence of fibroadenomas. Risk is also increased for those with more wealth as measured by either income or monthly rental. Furthermore, women with more years of education are more likely to have had a fibroadenoma excised. Although it is possible that the positive association of fibroadenoma and wealth could be due to environmental factors such as diet, a more likely explanation for the modest increase in risk is a heightened breast awareness among intelligent women, together with, in the United States, the ability to pay for medical advice and treatment.

**Table 9.1** Case control studies of reproductive factors and risk of fibroadenoma

| Author and year of study | Number of cases | Type of controls | Age at menarche | Nulliparity | Age at first pregnancy | Family history breast cancer |
|---|---|---|---|---|---|---|
| Sartwell, et al 1973[2] | 71 | Hospital | No effect | Relative risk 1.08 | No effect | Not mentioned |
| Kelsey, et al 1974[9] | 123 | Hospital | No effect | Relative risk 2.08 | No effect | No effect |
| Nomura, et al 1977[10] | 45 | Population | No effect | Relative risk 1.28 | No effect | Relative risk 2 |
| Cole, et al 1978[3] | 229 | Population | >12 – relative risk 1.7 | Slight effect | No effect | Not mentioned |
| Sartwell, et al 1978[5] | 155 | Hospital | Not mentioned | Relative risk 1.6 | >25 – relative risk 2.1 | Not mentioned |
| Ravnihar, et al 1979[11] | 95 | Hospital | No effect | Relative risk 1.25 | No effect | Slight |
| Soini, et al 1981[12] | 115 | Population | No effect | No effect | No effect | Not mentioned |
| Brinton, et al 1981[8] | 74 | Clinic | Not mentioned | No effect | No effect | Not mentioned |
| Parazzini, et al 1984[13] | 85 | Hospital | <14 – relative risk 1.5 | Relative risk 2.2 | No effect | Not mentioned |

**Table 9.2** Case control studies of social class, education, income, and risk of fibroadenoma

| Author and year of study | Social class | Income (US$) | Education (years) |
|---|---|---|---|
| Nomura, et al 1977[10] Relative risk | | <11,000  11,000 +<br>1.0      2.1 | <11  11–12  13 +<br>1.0  2.0    2.3 |
| Cole, et al 1978[3] Relative risk | | Monthly rental payment<br><100  100–124  175 +<br>1.0  1.4       1.0 | |
| Ravnihar, et al 1979[11] Relative risk | I    IV–V<br>1.5  0.84 | | <8  ≥12<br>0.96  1.34 |
| Soini, et al 1981[12] Relative risk | | | (University degree – 1.6) |
| Brinton, et al 1981[8] Relative risk | I    IV–V<br>1.0  0.44 | | |
| Fleming, et al 1982[4] Relative risk | I    IV–V<br>1.0  0.71 | | |
| Parazzini, et al 1984[13] Relative risk | | | <12 y  ≥12 y<br>1.0     1.0 |

*Oral contraception*

In the original study of Vessey *et al* which examined oral contraception and benign breast problems, it was found that there was an under-representation of women with fibroadenomas among the pill takers.[14] Accordingly, it was postulated that oral contraception might protect against fibroadenoma. A subsequent survey of physicians' attitudes, however, suggested that many believed that a past history of a breast lump was a relative contraindication to oral contraception and thus a selection bias may have been responsible for the original finding.[15] Subsequent studies from the United States and England have shown a slight apparent protective effect,[2, 8, 9] whereas results from Slovenia and Italy showed no effect Table 9.3.[11, 13, 16] There is certainly no evidence that oral contraception induces growth of fibroadenomas, and there is no reason why a young woman who has had a fibroadenoma excised – or managed conservatively with cytological confirmation – should not take oral contraceptives.

*Endocrine factors*

It has been reported that patients with fibroadenomas have a low urinary ratio of oestriol to oestradiol and oestrone[17] but others have found no difference between oestradiol concentrations in patients and controls.[18] Fibroadenoma cases and controls had normal urinary concentrations of pregnanediol.[19, 20] Sitruk-Ware and Martin reported low plasma progesterone concentrations in patients with fibroadenomas and have used topical progesterone treatment for women with benign breast lumps. The relationship of luteal phase insufficiency to the aetiology of fibroadenomas requires further investigation. A low progesterone concentration may not necessarily be an aetiological factor in the development of fibroadenomas, as most women with this problem will be young. It has been found that anovulatory cycles are a frequent occurrence in young women during the early years of menstruation.[21] No abnormalities of either basal concentrations of prolactin or concentrations of prolactin stimulated by thyrotrophin releasing

**Table 9.3** Oral contraceptives and risk of fibroadenomas

| Author and year of study | Relative risk |
|---|---|
| Vessey, *et al* 1972[14] | 0.43 |
| Sartwell, *et al* 1975[2] | 1.19 |
| Kelsey, *et al* 1978[9] | 0.93 |
| Ravnihar, *et al* 1979[11] | 1.0 |
| Brinton, *et al* 1981[8] | 0.35 |
| Parazzini, *et al* 1984[13] | 1.5 |
| Franceschi, *et al* 1984[16] | 1.0 |
| Mean | 0.91 |
| 95% confidence interval | 0.61 to 1.21 |

hormone have been found in plasma from patients with fibroadenomas,[22, 23] nor has any androgenic abnormality been detected.[24]

*Methylxanthines*

Increased concentrations of cyclic adenosine monophosphate (AMP) and cyclic guanosine monophosphate have been found within breast cancers and it has been suggested that caffeine, as an inhibitor of cyclic AMP phosphodiesterase, might further enhance this.[25] Minton *et al*[26] found increased concentrations of cyclic AMP in fibroadenomas compared with normal or fibrotic tissue, but this could have been attributable to increased cellularity within fibroadenomas. Boyle *et al*[27] conducted a case control study looking at a variety of benign conditions. They examined the risk of fibroadenomas in relationship to consumption of caffeine. There was no significant alteration in the odds ratio of women who consumed less than 30 mg, 31–250 mg, 251–500 mg, or more than 500 mg/day of caffeine. Thus it is unlikely that caffeine consumption plays any role in the aetiology of fibroadenomas.

## Fibroadenoma and risk of breast cancer

Those studies in which a relative risk of malignancy have been calculated for patients with histologically proven fibroadenomas are summarised in Table 9.4.[28-32] The original work of Donnelly *et al* found no significant increase in relative risk.[28] In contrast, Kodlin *et al* found a sevenfold increase in relative risk for women with fibroadenomas, with 16 observed cases in a population of 849 in which the expected number was 2.3.[29] Kodlin *et al* also reported that cases with higher scores of atypia had an increased risk, but did not separately analyse atypia scores within the fibroadenoma group. Thus one possible explanation for this unusually high relative risk might have been an over-representation of patients with atypical hyperplasia in the fibroadenoma group. Certainly, in the study of Page *et al*,[30] no increase in relative risk was found for women with fibroadenomas in which there was no evidence of atypical hyperplasia. Hutchinson *et al* reported a relative risk of

**Table 9.4**  Fibroadenoma and risk of breast cancer

| Author and year of study | Number of patients | Relative risk | 95% confidence interval |
|---|---|---|---|
| Donnelly, *et al* 1975[28] | 100 | 1.66 | 0.9  to 2.7 |
| Kodlin, *et al* 1977[29] | 849 | 7 | 6.26 to 7.74 |
| Page, *et al* 1978[30] | 189 | 1.25 | |
| Hutchinson, *et al* 1980[31] | 286 | 2.5 | 1.3  to 4.3 |
|    Fibroadenoma and fibrocystic disease | 164 | 0.9 | 0.11 to 3.2 |
|    Fibroadenoma, no fibrocystic disease | 122 | 3.82 | 1.83 to 7.03 |
| Roberts, *et al* 1984[32] | 138 | 0 | |

2.5 for all fibroadenomas,[31] but when these were subdivided into those with and without fibrocystic disease, the relative risks were 3.8 and 0.9, respectively. Roberts *et al* did not find any cases of malignancy on follow up of their patients with fibroadenomas.[32] Taken together these studies suggest that a fibroadenoma *per se* does not carry an increased risk of malignancy, but that any risk is conveyed by the presence of atypical change in surrounding breast tissue.

## Fibrocystic disease

Clinicians sometimes use the term 'fibrocystic disease' to describe patients with lumpy or painful breasts. The syndrome is also described as fibroadenosis but it may not be accompanied by the histological abnormalities of fibrocystic change as described below. The histopathological diagnosis of fibrocystic disease should be made only when the following are identified: microcysts, adenosis, apocrine metaplasia, gross cysts, epithelial hyperplasia, sclerosing adenosis, papillomatosis, a single papilloma, or atypical lobular hyperplasia. The changes may be present singly, but more usually in combination. Only patients who have these particular changes confirmed histologically will be considered in this section; women with gross cysts treated by aspiration will be discussed separately.

## Risk factors for fibrocystic disease

### Age

Fibrocystic disease is usually diagnosed in a slightly older age group than those with fibroadenoma with a peak incidence between the ages of 35 and 44, and a progressive reduction in incidence after the menopause. The age distribution of cases of fibrocystic disease from four studies[2-5] is given in Fig. 9.1.

### Weight

Four case control studies have examined the influence of weight on the diagnosis of biopsied fibrocystic disease.[3, 8, 11, 13] These have all shown a consistent reduction in relative risk for obese women (relative risk – 0.61, 95% confidence interval 0.51 to 0.73). This probably has a similar explanation to the observed inverse relationship between weight and diagnosis of fibroadenoma, because of the difficulty of detecting discrete lumps in the breasts of obese women. This contrasts with breast cancer in which the lump will almost always eventually become clinically apparent, and thus it has been found that obese postmenopausal women are at increased risk of breast cancer.

### Reproductive features

Fibrocystic disease predominantly affects premenopausal women, with a relative risk of 1.5 for premenopausal compared with postmenopausal

**Table 9.5** Case control studies of reproductive factors and risk of fibrocystic disease

| Author and year of study | Number of cases | Type of controls | Age at menarche | Nulliparity | Age at first pregnancy | Family history breast cancer |
|---|---|---|---|---|---|---|
| Sartwell, et al 1973[2] | 306 | Hospital | No effect | No effect | No effect | Not mentioned |
| Kelsey, et al 1974[9] | 209 | Hospital | No effect | Relative risk 1.94 | No effect >21 years – relative risk 1.9 | No effect Relative risk 2 |
| Nomura, et al 1977[10] | 275 | Population | No effect | Relative risk 1.5 | | Not mentioned |
| Cole, et al 1978[3] | 642 | Population | No effect | Slight effect | No effect | Not mentioned |
| Sartwell, et al 1978[5] | 783 | Hospital | Not mentioned | Relative risk 1.1 | >25 relative risk 1.7 | Not mentioned |
| Ravnihar, et al 1979[11] | 266 | Hospital | No effect | Relative risk 1.7 | No effect | Relative risk 1.88 |
| Soini, et al 1981[12] | 642 | Population | No effect | No effect | No effect | Not mentioned |
| Brinton, et al 1981[8] | 211 | Clinic | Not mentioned | No effect | No effect | Not mentioned |
| Parazzini, et al 1984[13] | 203 | Hospital | <14 relative risk 1.3 | Relative risk 1.6 | >30 – relative risk 2.6 | Not mentioned |

women. Thus it would be expected that its aetiology might be related to reproductive features with possible alterations in risk for nulliparous women or those who had a late first pregnancy or early menarche. This is not the case, however, and Table 9.5 shows that age at menarche, nulliparity, and age at first pregnancy do not significantly affect the risk of biopsied fibrocystic disease.

## Family history of breast cancer

Kelsey *et al*[9] found that a family history of breast cancer did not increase the risk of fibrocystic disease. In contrast, both Nomura *et al*[10] and Ravnihar *et al*[11] found a doubling of relative risk. It has not been determined whether this does represent a true linkage between breast cancer and fibrocystic disease, or merely arises because women with a family history are more likely to consult doctors about their breast problems. Furthermore, surgeons may be more reluctant to leave unbiopsied an equivocal area of lumpiness within the breast of a women who has a first degree relative with breast cancer.

## Endocrine factors

No consistent abnormalities of oestrogen, androgen, and prolactin secretion have been detected in patients with biopsy proved fibrocystic disease.[33] Although it has been reported that women with fibrocystic disease have raised plasma oestradiol concentrations during the luteal phase,[34] most studies have not found this abnormality.[35-38] Similarly, luteal phase progesterone deficiency found by some workers[18, 38] has not been confirmed by others.[39, 40] Subnormal plasma androgen concentrations have been reported in some patients with fibrocystic disease,[41, 42] but yet again others have not demonstrated any alteration,[43, 44] and Secreto *et al* have reported high concentrations of urinary androstanediol.[45]

Although baseline blood prolactin concentrations have been generally found to be normal in women with fibrocystic disease,[46-48] a consistently higher concentration after TRH stimulation with thyrotrophin releasing hormone has been reported.[49-51]

## Socio-economic factors

As with fibroadenomas, it has been found that women with biopsied fibrocystic disease are more likely to be wealthy, live in expensive houses, be better educated, and be members of social class 1. The results are summarised in Table 9.6. These findings are almost certainly not the result of any biological differences in richer women but because they are more likely to consult their doctors with breast lumps.

## Oral contraception

All the case-control studies which have examined oral contraception usage

**Table 9.6** Case control studies of social class, education, income, and risk of fibrocystic disease

| Author and year of study | Social class | | Income (US$) | | | | Education (years) | | |
|---|---|---|---|---|---|---|---|---|---|
| Nomura, et al 1977[10] | | | <11,000 | 11,000 + | | | <11 | 11–12 | 13 + |
| Relative risk | | | 1.0 | 1.6 | | | 1.0 | 1.5 | 1.7 |
| Cole, et al 1978[3] | | | Monthly rental payment | | | | | | |
| | | | <100 | 100–124 | 125–175 | 175 + | | | |
| Relative risk | | | 1.0 | 1.0 | 1.3 | 1.4 | | | |
| Ravnihar, et al 1979[11] | I | IV–V | | | | | | | |
| Relative risk | 1.12 | 2.1 | | | | | | | |
| Soini, et al 1981[12] | | | | | | | <8 y | ≥12 y | |
| Relative risk | | | | | | | 0.74 | 1.09 | |
| Brinton, et al 1981[8] | I | IV–V | | | | | (University degree 1.3) | | |
| Relative risk | 1.0 | 0.82 | | | | | | | |
| Parazzini, et al 1984[13] | I | IV–V | | | | | | | |
| Relative risk | 1.0 | 0.8 | | | | | | | |

**Table 9.7**   Oral contraceptives and relative risk of biopsied fibrocystic disease (ever versus never) modified from La Vecchia 1985[52]

| Author and year of study | Relative risk |
|---|---|
| Vessey, *et al* 1972[14] | 0.75 |
| Sartwell, *et al* 1973[2] | 0.87 |
| Kelsey, *et al* 1978[9] | 0.78 |
| Ravnihar, *et al* 1979[11] | 0.64 |
| Brinton, *et al* 1981[8] | 0.66 |
| Duffy, *et al* 1983[53] | 0.94 |
| Parazzini, *et al* 1984[13] | 0.86 |
| Franceschi, *et al* 1984[16] | 1.0 |
| Mean | 0.78 |
| 95% confidence interval | 0.67 to 0.91 |

and fibrocystic disease have recently been reviewed,[52] and have shown a decreasing risk of fibrocystic disease among pill takers (Table 9.7). The most recent study from Milan did not show any overall reduction in risk for users of oral contraceptives, but did show an apparent reduction in risk for long term use.[16] Because of the small numbers, however, the confidence intervals were wide.

There is a paradox in that although oral contraceptive usage reduces the incidence of fibrocystic disease it does not affect breast cancer incidence, either positively or negatively. Because of this, LiVolsi *et al* studied the histology of women having biopsies for benign conditions.[54] They found that marked atypia was as frequent in biopsies from women who were both users and non-users of the pill. Minimal or moderate atypia, however, was less frequently present among oral contraceptive users. Fasal and Paffenbarger examined the relationship between pill usage, benign breast disease, and risk of malignancy, and reported a relative risk of 11 for women who had had a prior breast biopsy for benign disease and had taken the pill for more than 6 years.[55] In subsequent studies, however, this apparent chance finding was not found to be a constant risk factor.[56]

*Methylxanthines*

In a case control study of discordant twins it was found that there was a significant positive association between caffeine consumption and risk of biopsied fibrocystic disease.[57] Boyle *et al* studied the relationship between caffeine consumption and the degree of hyperplasia and atypia in benign breast biopsies.[27] A dose response effect was observed in terms of caffeine intake and evidence of fibrocystic disease. Women consuming less than 30 mg of caffeine/day were assigned a risk ratio of 1, which increased to 1.5 for those taking 31–250 mg/day, 2 for 251–500 mg, and 2.3 for women reporting a intake of greater than 500 mg of caffeine/day. When the subgroup who were found to have atypical lobular hyperplasia were analysed, there was also a dose response effect, with a fivefold increase in risk for atypical lobular hyperplasia among those consuming more than 500 mg/day compared with those taking less than 30 mg. This work needs to be extended, as it raises the worrying possibility that large intakes of caffeine might increase the risk of premalignant atypical change which might not manifest as invasive malignancy until after a long latency period.

## Fibrocystic disease and breast cancer

Arguments have been advanced suggesting either no link between fibrocystic disease and malignancy or, alternatively, implicating the condition as being premalignant. Many of the follow up studies have been flawed by inclusion of too few cases, or by insufficient follow up, or by lack of histological characterisation of the condition, or by the absence of calculation of relative risk because expected numbers of cases within the population were not estimated. The situation has recently been reviewed by Webber and Boyd who ranked the cohort studies that had been carried out.[58] There were nine studies[28-31, 59-63] which did meet the minimum necessary requirements and the results of these are given in Table 9.8. These show a consistent increase in relative risk for those with fibrocystic disease, with mean of 2·8 (95% confidence interval 1.9 to 3.7).

The studies of Page *et al* and Hutchinson *et al* have dissected fibrocystic change into its component parts.[30, 31] It has been found that the cancer risk was doubled in women with epithelial hyperplasia and quadrupled in the presence of atypical epithelial hyperplasia, and that the risk was further increased by a first degree family history of malignancy.[64]

Thus it is now established that fibrocystic disease as a histological entity

**Table 9.8**   Biopsied fibrocystic disease and risk of breast cancer: cohort studies

| Author and year of study | Number of patients | Length of follow up (years) | Relative risk | 95% confidence intervals |
|---|---|---|---|---|
| Warren 1940[59] | 534 | 9 | 4.5 | 3.0 to 6.4 |
| Clagett, *et al* 1944[60] | 265 | 8 | 5.3 | 1.9 to 9.9 |
| Davis, *et al* 1964[61] | 317 | 13 | 1.7 | 0.7 to 3.7 |
| Veronesi and Pizzocaro 1968[62] | 1051 | 8 | 2 | 1.3 to 3.0 |
| Donnelly, *et al* 1975[28] | 96 | 30 | 2.9 | 2.2 to 3.6 |
| Monson, *et al* 1976[63] | 733 | 30 | 2.5 | 1.9 to 3.5 |
| Kodlin, *et al* 1977[29] | 1106 | 7 | 2.8 | 1.8 to 3.3 |
| Page, *et al* 1978[30] | 925 | 16 | 1.4 | 0.9 to 2.0 |
| Hutchinson, *et al* 1980[31] | 1053 | 13 | 2.1 | 1.6 to 2.7 |
| | | Mean | 2.8 | 1.9 to 3.7 |

does not convey any increased risk of breast cancer unless moderate to severe hyperplasia, with or without atypia, is present. To place atypical lobular hyperplasia in context as a risk factor for breast cancer, it was found that the combination of it with family history of breast cancer was present in only 39 out of 10 366 women (0.004%).

## Gross cystic disease

Patients with gross cystic disease – that is, palpable breast cysts treated by either aspiration or excision – show a variant of fibrocystic change. Nowadays most of such cases are treated by aspiration alone. Provided that the lump disappears, the aspirate is not blood-stained, and the cyst does not recur, these patients are usually treated and then discharged. Are such patients at any greater risk of malignancy than other women with biopsy proven fibrocystic disease? Do women with gross cysts share risk factors with breast cancer patients? This latter question has been addressed by Duffy *et al* who compared 188 women who had proven gross cysts with 2213 asymptomatic controls.[53] Predictably, cysts occurred more frequently in the premenopausal group (relative risk 1.45). There was no increase in risk for parity, lactation, family history of breast cancer, or contraceptive use among the cyst group. Patients with gross cysts were more likely to have had previous breast complaints (relative risk 2.4) or a prior breast biopsy (relative risk 7.1).

## Gross cysts and breast cancer

Approximately 1% of patients presenting with breast cysts are found to have carcinoma masquerading as a cyst.[65, 66] When these cases are excluded there does not appear to be any short term increased risk of breast carcinoma. Nevertheless, the careful follow up study by Haagensen has shown that women with gross cysts have an approximate three fold increase in life time risk of subsequent malignancy.[67] This is remarkably similar to the overall risk which has been reported for fibrocystic disease, and does suggest that the histological premalignant changes of atypical lobular or ductal hyperplasia are as likely to be associated with fibrocystic disease with microcysts as with gross cystic disease.

## Mastalgia

Various classifications of varying complexity have been proposed for women presenting with breast pain.[68, 69] Probably the simplest division of cases is into those with either cyclical mastalgia or non-cyclical mastalgia of extramammary or intramammary type.[70] The commonest problem is cyclical mastalgia, which is usually a self limiting condition. There are however, a few patients with severe persistent pain who do ask for treatment. Taking the combined results from five prospective clinical trials on patients with mastalgia, the mean age at presentation was 37 years.[71-75] By definition, the condition affects premenopausal women, although there may be an over-representation of women who have previously had hysterectomies. No case control studies have specifically compared women suffering from severe mastalgia needing treatment, with age and parity matched controls. The influence of socioeconomic status is unknown and no international comparisons been conducted. Within Britain there may be regional differences between the incidence rates of mastalgia.

## Endocrine background

A condition which tends to worsen during the luteal phase of the menstrual cycle is most likely to be the result of some abnormality of hypophyseal or ovarian function. No consistent abnormalities have been found, however, in oestradiol or progesterone or prolactin concentrations among women with mastalgia. Nevertheless studies using stimulation tests have shown that prolactin release is significantly increased in most women with cyclical mastalgia.[51]

Despite the lack of identifiable endocrine dysfunction, a variety of hormonal manipulations have been found to relieve mastalgia including the antigonadotrophin drug danazol, the prolactin inhibitor bromocriptine, and – more recently – the antioestrogen, tamoxifen. Approximately half the patients will relapse within three months of discontinuing treatment, however, suggesting that for many patients the underlying endocrine problem is not permanently altered by hormonal therapy.

## Methylxanthines and mastalgia

The relationship between methylxanthines, in particular caffeine, and breast pain is still under investigation. Minton *et al*[76] originally reported that among a group of women with mastalgia who stopped taking caffeine there was complete or partial improvement in 98%. Among those who reduced their intake mastalgia was relieved in 75%, compared with only 25% of those whose caffeine intake was unchanged. Brooks *et al*[77] also reported that among 66 women who restricted their caffeine intake, there was an overall reduction in pain in 92%. This concept of caffeine reduction has been subjected to a prospective controlled randomised trial by Ernster *et al*[78] in which patients changed to a caffeine restricted diet or continued with their usual diet. They found a statistically significant reduction in clinically palpable breast findings but expressed reservation about whether this was clinically relevant. Breast pain was not directly measured, but the authors reported their impression that there was a reduction in tenderness among the group receiving a caffeine free diet. Heyden and Muhlbaier[79] followed up a group of patients with mastalgia in whom there was no reduction in caffeine intake, and reported that breast pain spontaneously disappeared in 31%.

The drug theophylline is a more powerful inhibitor of phosphodiesterase than caffeine and thus any effect on mastalgia should be more pronounced among women taking this drug for asthma. Hindi-Alexander *et al*[80] studied a group of asthmatic women (62 receiving theophylline), a control group of allergic women (66 not receiving theophylline) and another control group of non-allergic, non-asthmatic women. The mean severity of fibrocystic breast disease (largely measured by pain and tenderness) was similar for the three groups during the period of the study. Nevertheless there was a relationship between severity of symptoms and methylxanthine intake which became more significant after controlling for age, menopause, and parity.

In a recent controlled trial Allen and Froberg[81] randomised patients with mastalgia to three groups: caffeine free diet (n = 18), cholesterol free diet (n = 19), and a controlled normal diet (n = 19). These remained from a total of 118 patients originally entered into the study. There was no change in the mean pain or tenderness score for any of the three groups throughout the four months of the trial. The authors did, however, conduct a follow up telephone questionnaire of 39 of the 56 women who completed the study; 36% said that they had reduced their caffeine intake during the trial period and 25% of these reported a reduction in breast pain. 10 out of 39 (26%) increased their caffeine intake and 30% of these complained of more breast pain.

Thus evidence implicating caffeine in mastalgia is largely anecdotal, partly because few authors have used linear analogue scoring to determine individual changes in breast pain. This subject warrants further study by prospective randomised trials.

## Mastalgia and malignancy

Although a few patients with non-palpable breast cancers will present with breast pain, for the majority the pain will be the reason for carrying out mammography which identifies the non-palpable lesion.[82] Overall approximately 10% of patients with breast cancer will have some breast pain, compared with approximately 30% of symptomatic women attending breast clinics. To date there is no compelling evidence of a relationship between mastalgia and malignancy.

## Conclusions

Review of published reports reveals that the use of the phrase 'benign breast disease' has seriously inhibited progress in the understanding of a variety of benign breast conditions. The lumping together of patients with fibroadenomas, fibrocystic change, and cyclical mastalgia has led to a blurring of any abnormalities that may exist within these individual groups of patients. The relationship between various benign conditions and malignancy is now becoming much more clear, and most patients who have had breast biopsies for benign conditions carry no increased life long risk of malignancy. A few histologically identifiable patients do have an increased risk, and these particular patients do warrant long term follow up. For most women, however, anxiety can be allayed, and following this they do not require any closer surveillance than their non-biopsied neighbours.

## References

1. Cant PJ, Madden MV, Close PM, *et al.* Case for conservative management of selected fibroadenomas of the breast. *Br J Surg* 1987; **74**: 857–59.
2. Sartwell PE, Arthes FG, Tonascia JA. Benign and malignant tumours : lack of association with oral contraceptive use. *N Engl J Med* 1973; **22**: 551–54.
3. Cole P, Elwood JM, Kaplan SD. Incidence rates and risk factors of benign breast neoplasms. *Am J Epidemiol* 1978; **108**: 112–20.
4. Fleming NT, Armstrong BK, Sheiner HJ. The comparative epidemiology of benign breast lumps and breast cancer in Western Australia. *Int J Cancer* 1982; **30**: 147–52.
5. Sartwell PE, Arthes FG, Tonascia JA. Benign and malignant breast tumours : epidemiologic similarities. *Int J Epidemiol* 1978; **7**: 217–21.
6. Frantz VK, Pickren JW, Melcher GW, Auchinloss H. Incidence of chronic cystic disease in so called 'normal breasts'. A study based on 225 post-mortem examinations. *Cancer*. 1951; **4**: 762–83.
7. Holmberg L, Adami H-O, Persson I, *et al.* Demands on surgical inpatient services after mass mammographic screening. *Br Med J* 1986; **293**: 779–82.
8. Brinton LA, Vessey MP, Flavel R, Yeates D. Risk factors for benign breast disease. *Am J Epidemiol* 1981; **113**: 203–14.
9. Kelsey JL, Lindfors KK, White, C. A case-control study of the epidemiology of benign breast diseases with reference to oral contraceptive use. *Int J Epidemiol* 1974; **3**: 333–40.
10. Nomura A, Comstock GW, Tonascia JA. Epidemiologic characteristics of benign breast disease. *Am J Epidemiol* 1977; **105**: 505–12.
11. Ravnihar B, Seigel DG, Lindtner J. An epidemiologic study of breast cancer and benign breast neoplasms in relation to oral contraceptive and oestrogen use. *European Journal of Cancer* 1979; **15**: 395–405.
12. Soini I, Aine R, Lauslahti K, Hakama M. Independent risk factors of benign and malignant breast lesions. *Am J Epidemiol* 1981; **114**: 507–14.
13. Parazzini F, La Vecchia C, Franceschi S, *et al.* Risk factors for pathologically confirmed benign breast disease. *Am J Epidemiol* 1984; **120**: 115–22.
14. Vessey MP, Doll R, Sutton PM. Oral contraceptives and breast neoplasia : a retrospective study. *Br Med J* 1972; **3**: 719–24.
15. Janerich DT, Glevatis DM, Dugan JM. Benign breast disease and oral contraceptive use. *JAMA* 1977; **237**: 2199–201.
16. Franceschi S, La Vecchia C, Parazzini F, *et al.* Oral contraceptives and benign breast disease : a case-control study. *Am J Obstet Gynecol* 1984; **149**: 602–06.
17. Serban MD, Stroe E, Klepsch I, *et al.* Data hormonale in mastopatii. *Studii Cercetari Endocrinologica* 1963; **14**: 399–408.
18. Sitruk-Ware LR, Sterkers N, Mowszowicz I, Mauvais-Jarvis P. Inadequate corpus luteum function in women with benign breast disease. *J Clin Endocrinol Metab* 1977; **44**: 771–74.
19. Marmoston J, Crowley LG, Myers SM, *et al.* Urinary excretion of estrone, estradiol and estriol by patients with breast cancer and benign breast disease. *Am J Obstet Gynecol* 1965; **92**: 460–67.
20. Martin PM, Kuttenn F, Serment H, Mauvais-Jarvis P. Studies on clinical, hormonal and pathological correlations in breast fibroadenomas. *J Steroid Biochem* 1978; **9**: 1251–55.
21. Apter D, Viinikka L, Vihko R. Hormonal pattern of adolescent menstrual cycles. *J Clin Endocrinol Metab* 1978; **47**: 944–54.
22. Franchimont P, Dourcy C, Legros JJ, *et al.* Dosage de la prolactine dans les conditions hormones et pathologiques. *Ann Endocrinol* 1976; **37**: 127–56.

23. Ohgo S, Kato Y, Chihara K, Imura H. Plasma prolactin responses to thyrotropin-releasing hormone in patients with breast cancer. *Cancer* 1976; **37**: 1412–16.
24. Marmoston J, Crowley LG, Myers SM, *et al*. Urinary excretion of neutral 17-Ketosteroids and pregnanediol of patients with breast cancer and benign breast disease. *Am J Obstet Gynecol* 1965; **92**: 447–59.
25. Minton JP, Matthews RH, Wisenbaugh TW. Elevated levels of 3'5' cyclic monophosphate levels in human and animal tumours in vivo. *JNCI* 1976; **57**: 39–41.
26. Minton JP, Foecking MK, Webster DJT, Matthews RH. Caffeine cyclic nucleotides and breast disease. *Surgery* 1979; **86**: 105–08.
27. Boyle CA, Berkowitz GS, LiVolsi VA, *et al*. Caffeine consumption and fibrocystic disease : a case-control epidemiological study. *JNCI* 1984; **72**: 1015–19.
28. Donnelly PK, Baker KW, Carney JA, O'Fallon WM. Benign breast lesions and subsequent breast carcinomas in Rochester, Minnesota. *Mayo Clin Proc* 1975; **50**: 650–56.
29. Kodlin D, Winger EE, Morgenstern NL, Chen V. Chronic mastopathy and breast cancer. *Cancer* 1977; **39**: 2603–07.
30. Page DL, Vander Zwagg R, Rogers LW, *et al*. Relation between component parts of fibrocystic disease and breast cancer. *JNCI* 1978; **61**: 1055–63.
31. Hutchinson WB, Thomas DB, Hamlin WB, *et al*. Risk of breast cancer in women with benign breast disease. *JNCI* 1980; **65**: 13–20.
32. Roberts MM, Jones V, Elton RA, *et al*. Risk of breast cancer in women with history of benign disease of the breast. *Br Med J* 1984; **288**: 275–78.
33. Wang DY, Fentiman IS. Epidemiology and endocrinology of benign breast disease. *Breast Cancer Res Treat* 1985; **6**: 5–36.
34. England PC, Skinner LG, Cottrell KM, Sellwood RA. Serum oestradiol-17 beta in women with benign and malignant breast disease. *Br J Cancer* 1974; **30**: 571–76.
35. Swain MC, Hayward JL, Bulbrook RD. Plasma oestradiol and progesterone in benign breast disease. *European Journal of Cancer* 1973; **9**: 553–56.
36. Golinger RC, Krebs J, Fisher ER, Danowski TS. Hormones and the pathophysiology of fibrocystic mastopathy. Elevated luteinising hormone levels. *Surgery* 1978; **84**: 212–15.
37. Bagli NP, Shah PN, Mistry SS. The estriol quotient in fibrocystic disease, a high risk group for breast cancer. *Indian J Cancer* 1980; **17**: 201–04.
38. DeBoever J, Vanderkerhove D. Benign breast disease : steroid concentrations. *J Steroid Biochem* 1982; Abstract 338
39. England PC, Skinner LG, Cottrell KM, Sellwood RA. Sex hormones in breast disease. *Br J Surg* 1975; **62**: 806–09.
40. Walsh PV, Wang DY, McDicken I, *et al*. Serum progesterone concentration during the luteal phase in women with benign breast disease. *Eur J Cancer Clin Oncol* 1984; **20**: 1339–43.
41. Brennan MJ, Bulbrook RD, Deshpande N, *et al*. Urinary and plasma androgens in benign breast disease. *Lancet* 1973; i: 1076–79.
42. Gorlich M, Heise E, Pradja N, Hindy I. The excretion of 17-ketosteroids in patients suffering from mastopathia fibrocystica and mammary carcinoma. *Arch Geschwulstforsch* 1975; **45**: 648–57.
43. Wang DY, Hayward JL, Bulbrook RD. Testosterone levels in the plasma of normal women and patients with benign breast disease or breast cancer. *European Journal of Cancer* 1966; **2**: 373–76.
44. Jones MK, Dyer GI, Ramsay ID, Collins WP. Studies on apparent free cortisol

and testosterone in plasma from patients with breast tumours. *Br J Cancer* 1977; **35**: 885–87.

45. Secreto G, Fariselli G, Bandieramonte G, *et al*. Androgen excretion in women with a family history of breast cancer or with epithelial hyperplasia or cancer of the breast. *Eur J Cancer Clin Oncol* 1983; **19**: 5–10.

46. Boyns AR, Cole EN, Griffiths K, *et al*. Plasma prolactin in breast cancer. *European Journal of Cancer* 1973; **9**: 99–102.

47. Malarkey WB, Schroeder LL, Stevens VC, *et al*. Disordered nocturnal prolactin regulation in women with breast cancer. *Cancer Res* 1977; **37**: 4650–54.

48. Sheth NA, Ranadive KJ, Suraiya JN, Sheth AR. Circulating levels of prolactin in human breast cancer. *Br J Cancer* 1975; **32**: 160–67.

49. Ofuji N, Ogawa N, Miyoshi M, *et al*. Plasma prolactin and thyroid stimulating hormone in patients with breast cancer. *Folia Endocrinologica Japonica* 1976; **52**: 565–71.

50. Geller S, Grenier J, Nahoul K, Scholler R. Insuffisance lutéale et mastopathies bénignes. Etude à la lumier des données de l'épreuve combinée LH-RH + TRH couplée a l'étude des stéroides ovaries. *Ann Endocrinol* 1979; **40**: 45–46.

51. Kumar S, Mansel RE, Scanlon MF, Hughes LF. Secretory response of prolactin and TSH in benign breast disease and after TRH stimulation. *Br J Surg* 1983; **70**: 293–95.

52. La Vecchia CL, Parazzini F, Franceschi S, Decarli A. Risk factors for benign breast disease and their relation with breast cancer risk. Pooled information from epidemiologic studies. *Tumori* 1985; **71**: 167–78.

53. Duffy SW, Roberts MM, Elton RA. Risk factors relevant to cystic breast disease: a case control study. *J Epidemiol Community Health* 1983; **37**: 271–73.

54. LiVolsi VA, Stadel BV, Kelsey JL, *et al*. Fibrocystic breast disease in oral contraceptive users. A histopathological evaluation of epithelial atypia. *N Engl J Med* 1978; **299**: 381–85.

55. Fasal E, Paffenbarger RS. Oral contraceptives as related to cancer and benign lesions of the breast. *JNCI* 1975; **55**: 767–73.

56. Paffenbarger RS, Kampert JB, Chang H. Oral contraceptives and breast cancer risk. *Les Editions de L'INSERM* 1979; **83**: 93–114.

57. Odennheimer DJ, Zunzunegui MV, King MC, *et al*. Risk factors for benign breast disease : a case control study of discordant twins. *Am J Epidemiol* 1984; **120**: 565–71.

58. Webber W, Boyd N. A critique of the methodology of benign breast disease and breast cancer risk. *JNCI* 1986; **77** 397–404.

59. Warren S. The relation of chronic mastitis to carcinoma of the breast. *Surg Gynecol Obstet* 1940; **71**: 257–73.

60. Clagett OT, Plimpton NC, Root GT. Lesions of the breast. The relationship of benign lesions to carcinoma. *Surgery* 1944; **15**: 414–19.

61. Davis HH, Simons MA, Davis TB. Cystic disease of the breast : relationship to carcinoma. *Cancer* 1964; **17**: 957–78.

62. Veronesi U, Pizzocaro G. Breast cancer in women subsequent to cystic disease of the breast. *Surg Gynecol Obstet* 1968; **126**: 529–32.

63. Monson RR, Yen S, McMahon B, Warren S. Chronic mastitis and carcinoma of the breast. *Lancet* 1976; **ii**: 224–26.

64. Dupont WD, Page DL. Risk factors for breast cancer in women with proliferative breast disease. *N Engl J Med* 1985; **312**: 146–51.

65. Hermann JB. Mammary cancer subsequent to aspiration of cysts in the breast. *Ann Surg* 1971; **133**: 40–43.

66. Devitt JE, Barr JR. The clinical recognition of cystic carcinoma of the breast. *Surg Gynecol Obstet* 1984; **159**: 130–32.

67. Haagensen CD. *Diseases of the Breast*. Philadelphia, WB Saunders, 1971.
68. Preece PE, Mansel RE, Bolton PM, *et al*. Clinical syndromes of mastalgia. *Lancet* 1976; ii 670–73.
69. Bishop HM, Blamey RW. A suggested classification of breast pain. *Postgrad Med J* 1979; **55**: 59–60.
70. Fentiman IS. Tamoxifen and mastalgia : an emerging indication. *Drugs* 1986; **32**: 477–80.
71. Mansel RE, Preece PE, Hughes LE. A double blind trial of the prolactin inhibitor bromocriptine in painful benign breast disease. *Br J Surg* 1978; **65**: 724–27.
72. Blichert-Toft M, Nyboe-Andersen A, Henriksen OB, Mygind T. Treatment of mastalgia with bromocriptine : a double blind cross-over study. *Br Med J* 1979; i: 237.
73. Gorins A, Ferret F, Tournant B, *et al*. A French double-blind cross-over study (danazol versus placebo) in the treatment of severe fibrocystic breast disease. *Eur J Gynaecol Oncol* 1984; **2**: 85–89.
74. Fentiman IS, Caleffi M, Brame K, *et al*. Double-blind controlled trial of tamoxifen therapy for mastalgia. *Lancet* 1986; i 287–88.
75. Powles TJ, Ford HT, Gazet JC. A randomised clinical trial to compare tamoxifen with danazol for treatment of benign mammary dysplasia. *Breast Disease-Senologia* 1987; **2**: 1–5.
76. Minton JP, Abou-Issa H, Reiches N, Roseman JM. Clinical and biochemical studies on methylxanthine-related fibrocystic breast disease. *Surgery* 1981; **90**: 299–303.
77. Brooks PG, Gart S, Heldfond AJ, *et al*. Measuring the effect of caffeine restriction on fibrocystic breast disease. *J Reprod Med* 1981; **26**: 279–82.
78. Ernster VL, Mason C, Goodson WH, *et al*. Effects of caffeine-free diet on benign breast disease : a randomised trial. *Surgery* 1984; **91**: 263–67.
79. Heyden S, Muhlbaier LH. Prospective study of fibrocystic breast disease and caffeine consumption. *Surgery*. 1984; **96**: 479–83.
80. Hindi-Alexander MC, Zielezny MA, Montes N, *et al*. Theophylline and fibrocystic breast disease. *J Allergy Clin Immunol* 1985; **75**: 709–15.
81. Allen SS, Froberg DG. The effect of decreased caffeine consumption on benign proliferative breast disease : a randomised clinical trial. *Surgery* 1987; **101**: 720–30.
82. Preece PE, Baum M, Mansel RE, *et al*. Importance of mastalgia in operable breast cancer. *Br Med J* 1982; **284**: 1299–1300.

# 10

# Operations for benign conditions of the breast: indications and techniques

The reasons for operating on benign lesions in the breast are: (a) for diagnosis, because the benign lesion cannot be distinguished from cancer without full histological examination, and (b) for discomfort or symptoms worrying to the patient.

## Operation for diagnostic reasons

In patients who present to the symptomatic referral clinic much the most common reason for operation is the finding of a solid lump; other reasons are nipple discharge, nipple eczema, or an impalpable mammographic abnormality. In women who have been referred from breast cancer screening units the latter reason predominates. In this chapter the management of a breast lump, and the investigation of nipple discharge and of nipple eczema are described.

## Operation for symptomatic reasons

The management of inflammatory lesions in the breast is described below. Breast pain which is unassociated with an inflammatory lesion is rarely a reason for operation. Most patients complaining of breast pain require only reassurance as to the nature of the pain, but occasionally pain and tenderness are severe enough to make a difference to a woman's life. Bad cyclical breast pain is treated by hormonal means, localised fibromyalgia syndrome (Tietze's syndrome) by local injection of hydrocortisone, and breast pain due to cervical spondylitis by physiotherapy. This leaves only one unusual pain, which we term 'trigger spot' – a single, tender area in the breast which has failed to respond to hydrocortisone injection. Here excision of the tender area has about a 50% expectation of relieving the pain.

## Management of a breast lump

The most common reason for presentation to the general practitioner is that a woman believes that she has a breast lump (table 10.1). The essential investigation for this or any other symptom is careful palpation of the breasts: the history is relatively unimportant.

Doctors working in the referral clinic must be fully confident of their skill in breast palpation. There are two useful guides which help to form the decision as to whether an abnormality is present or not. The first is that if on careful palpation the examiner decides that a lump is present, then he or she must not reverse that decision in the light of another investigation. For example, the examiner should not decide that there may be a cyst – attempt to aspirate – and then decide that as no fluid is withdrawn no lump is present; similarly a clinical decision that a lump is present should not be reversed by a mammogram which does not show the lump. The second guide is that the decision that a lump is present means that, unless the lump proves to be a cyst, a tissue diagnosis is required which may include operation; this realisation greatly sharpens the decision.

The ordering of a mammogram for investigation should mean that the examiner believes that no true lump is present but there is a 'lumpy' area in the breast requiring further investigation. In a recent survey at Nottingham City Hospital, in a five year period more than 5000 women were sent for mammography from the symptomatic clinic; 325 cancers were diagnosed in this period, in only nine would the diagnosis not have been reached without mammography, and four of these were cancers in the breast opposite to that of the complaint. Mammography is an excellent method for screening the breast but its use and interpretation in the symptomatic breast must be with caution.

Once the examiner has decided that a lump is present then an attempt at needle aspiration is made to determine whether the lump is a cyst. If this is so it is aspirated fully and the breast repalpated. As long as no residual lump is present the woman is reassured and discharged. Cysts are most common in the 40–50 age group, and rare under the age of 30 or in postmenopausal women; if they occur postmenopausally they should be further investigated as they may be associated with an intracystic or mucoid carcinoma.

If the lump is not cystic then either Trucut biopsy or fine needle aspiration

**Table 10.1**  Symptoms with which 1445 women were referred to the breast clinic

| | |
|---|---:|
| Breast lump or painful lump | 933 |
| Tender 'lumpy' areas | 110 |
| Breast pain | 224 |
| Nipple discharge | 75 |
| Nipple retraction | 36 |
| Nipple eczema | 3 |
| Swelling of breast | 7 |
| Other | 57 |

cytology is required. Trucut biopsy under local anaesthetic delivers a core suitable for histological examination by any trained pathologist. Some lumps, however, are too small and mobile or too hard for Trucut biopsy. A suitable specimen for analysis may be obtained in many of these by fine needle (23 g) aspiration. This technique requires a good specimen on the part of the clinician but particularly expertise in interpretation by the pathologist. The danger lies in the risk of making a false positive diagnosis of cancer; if the pathologist is not confident in his or her ability to avoid this then the technique should be abandoned and Trucut biopsy should be the outpatient method used in that hospital.

The procedure in many units after outpatient biopsy is, on receipt of a biopsy or cytology positive for cancer, to proceed to the definitive treatment of that cancer and to excise all other lumps for full histological examination. This leads to the removal of fibroadenomas, particularly in women aged 35 or under, and areas of fibrocystic disease in women aged 35 to 50. Other benign entities presenting as lumps are juvenile fibroadenoma (Fig. 10.1), sclerosing adenosis, sterile abscesses, and – rarely – lymph nodes or granulomatous conditions – tuberculosis, sarcoid, or granulomatous mastitis.

Although operative breast biopsy is a simple procedure it has two complications which are unfortunately only too common: the discomfort of a wound haematoma with (occasionally) superadded infection, and the production of unsightly scars.

Some solid benign lumps, particularly fibroadenomas, can be safely diagnosed without operation. In Nottingham we have tried to avoid unnecessary biopsy by setting strict protocols for the management of breast lumps. These are based upon the age of the patient (under 35 breast cancer is rare and becomes rarer the younger the patient), upon the clinical feel of the lump, upon fine needle aspiration cytology, and upon the appearance of the lump on imaging. Our present procedure with solid lumps that feel clinically benign in women under the age of 50 is first to offer the choice to the woman of leaving the lump alone or removing it. If she decides to leave the lump in the breast then the following criteria are applied:

- the lump must feel benign
- it must appear benign or be invisible on ultrasound and on mammography
- fine needle aspirations one week apart must show satisfactory numbers of entirely benign epithelial cells on cytology

As long as these criteria are fulfilled the lump is measured, checked by palpation, and measured again at three months and the patient then discharged. Under the age of 25 the criteria are more relaxed: only one fine needle aspiration is required and as long as the cytology shows no atypical cells there is no need for operation. Between 25 and 35 ultrasound alone is carried out for imaging as the breast is too dense for mammography below the age of 35.

If any one of the criteria is not met then excision-biopsy is strongly advised. Once a decision to remove the lump is made, the woman is admitted as soon as possible.

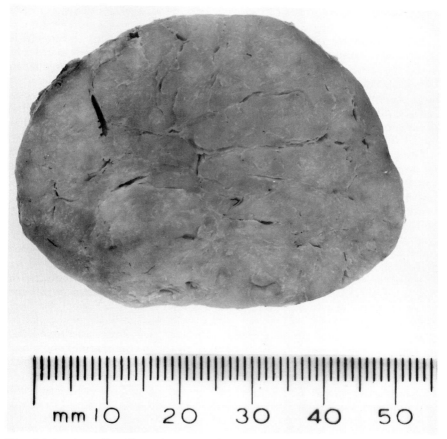

**Fig 10.1** Juvenile fibroadenoma: these present as large lesions (often 6–10 cm in diameter) in the breasts of women aged 18–22.

## Excision biopsy or incision biopsy of a breast lump

Breast biopsy under local anaesthetic can be uncomfortable and bleeding may be a problem. Unless the lump is at the periphery of the breast general anaesthetic is therefore preferred.

Day case biopsy is suitable. A number of rather indefinite edged lesions, thought to constitute a definite lump in the clinic, may not feel suspicious on the day of admission. The operating surgeon must examine the breast and if uncertain that a lump is present call for a re-evaluation by a senior member of the breast team; juniors should not feel obliged to operate unless they themselves are convinced that a lump is present.

The planned operation for a discrete lump is excision; that for a larger indefinite area is incision biopsy, taking a generous sized area from the centre of the mass. After skin incision a lump is not as easy to locate as beforehand, so it is worth placing an 18 or 21 gauge needle in the lump prior to incising the skin.

For the best cosmetic result the skin around the edge of the areola is marked in ink and a skin incision made just avoiding the pigment in order to avoid the rare complication of tatooing. Lumps 3–4 cm from the areola can be reached through such an incision by next dissecting subcutaneously with large straight blunt scissors. The plane between subcutaneous fat and breast fat is readily identified. If the lump is further from the areola, or is deep in the breast, the incision is made over the lump: I prefer circumferential incision paralled to the areola edge.

Once over the lump the superficial fascia is pushed aside and the deeper layers over the lump are reached. The inexperienced surgeon may again be caught unawares. The lump feels as though it is directly under the superficial fascia and the surgeon may try to seize it with tissue forceps. A smooth lump, however, such as a fibroadenoma, is lying deeper among the connective and epithelial tissue of the breast – this simply slips from the tissue forceps leaving the surgeon holding the wrong piece. The preferred approach is to incise the breast tissue vertically with a scalpel until the lump itself is reached (Fig. 10.2).

If there is no clearly defined lump at operation then incision is made to the centre of the mass and a piece of tissue about half an inch wide and encompassing the breadth of the main mass is cut out with a scalpel (incision-biopsy).

If there is a clear rounded lump – for example a fibroadenoma – the surgeon dissects close to this with a scalpel or sharp scissors until enough of the surface is exposed to seize the lump with tissue forceps, after which dissection close to the surface is completed.

Diathermy haemostasis is carried out throughout and a lengthy inspection and diathermy of the cavity is required. A suction drain is placed in all but the smallest and driest wounds and the skin is closed with interrupted 4.0 polypropylene (Prolene) sutures, which are replaced by Steristrips on the fourth day, or subcuticular 4.0 polyglycolic acid (Dexon).

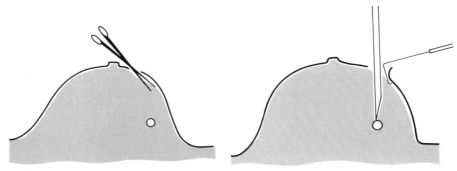

**Fig 10.2a&b**   The approach to a breast lump.

## The procedure of marker biopsy

'Marker biopsy' is our term for excision-biopsy of a mammographic abnormality without a palpable lump. A marker wire is placed in the breast using a steriotactic device which may be attached to some mammographic machines. This is easy to use and enables the wire to be placed with great accuracy thus limiting the extent of excision necessary for adequate diagnosis. The marker wire should be stout enough to be felt easily by the surgeon after incision within the breast tissue; the tip should engage firmly in the tissue. The Nottingham needle (Mediplus Ltd) fulfills these criteria.

The marker needle is placed in the breast under local anaesthetic (Fig. 10.3), with the needle parallel to the chest wall to avoid the marker wire being sucked in towards the chest should it come loose; the wire is bent to 90° at the point of entry to the skin, a piece of lead shot is pinched on to the wire at skin level and the wire taped to the skin. The position is checked by taking a lateral (Fig. 10.3(b) ) and a craniocaudal film.

The operation is carried out under general anaesthetic. A small circuma-reolar incision (about 3 cm long) is made over the point of the needle, which is estimated by measuring from the skin entry point on the two films. Subcutaneous dissection is carried out for several centimetres around the incision and up as far as the needle shaft just under the skin. The breast tissue is cut directly down with the scalpel so that the shaft of the needle is again encountered 1–2 cm above the tip. The shaft is grasped with artery forceps (old!) and the assistant holds the needle steady. The tip is now defined; sometimes a clear lesion can then be felt and is removed – if not, the tissue around the needle tip is excised by cutting with the scalpel down parallel to the needle on both sides and across about 1 cm below it. This tissue, including the needle tip, is then pulled upwards with tissue forceps and sharp dissection frees it from behind. A piece about 1.5 cm square is removed. This is immediately X-rayed which is best carried out with a machine designed for specimen X-ray (we use the Faxitron, Vinten Instruments). The processor dedicated for mammography is not required for the films which can be developed in the X-ray department if this is nearer to the operating theatre than the mammographic unit; for this the film is exposed at 20 kV for 7–9 seconds. The surgeon should mark the edges of the tissue with sutures for orientation.

Once the surgeon is satisfied that the biopsy taken is the lesion identified on X-ray then the tissue is sent for histological examination. The skin is sutured with a suction drain left in the cavity. Frozen section is not advised for these lesions, which require care and time for correct interpretation. The pathologist later uses the Faxitron machine to aid in the identification of the lesion by making several slices and X-raying these (Fig. 10.4).

## Nipple discharge

The patient complaining of a nipple discharge should first be questioned to ensure that, rather than a true nipple discharge, the complaint is not actually

a

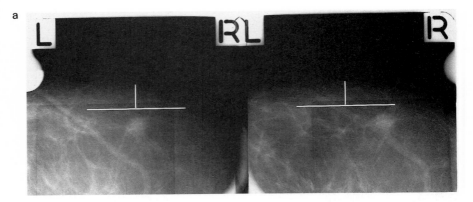

b

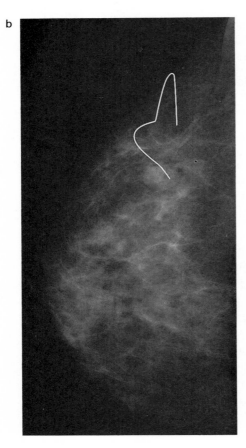

**Fig 10.3** Use of the steriotatic device fitted to a mammogram machine for localisation of an impalpable lesion. X-rays are taken with the machine inclined 15° either side of the perpendicular. The two views (3a) are placed in a viewer – marks set over the lesion and the adjustment to the medio/laterateral, vertical, and antero/posterior planes are shown. After adjustment of the machine the needle is fed down into the breast and accurately marks the lesion (3b).

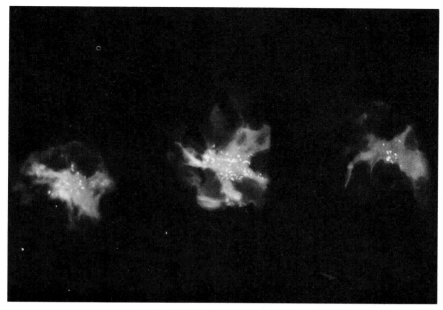

**Fig 10.4**   Specimen X-rays of slices prepared for histological examination.

of some staining on the bra or nightdress. This may arise from soreness of the nipple due to inflammation from retained secretions with an indrawn nipple, or to Paget's disease of the nipple.

The patient is examined – if a lump is found then the management becomes that of a lump (discussed above). If no lump is present an attempt is made to express the discharge, and the number of ducts involved is noted.

A multiduct discharge – which is frequently bilateral – may be regarded as an upset of physiology rather than a pathological entity. As long as the discharge is multiduct and the breast is otherwise clinically normal the woman needs only reassurance although mammography is an extra precaution. Occasionally such a discharge may be heavy and the patient wishes surgery for social reasons. The best operation is excision of the central ducts (see below).

About 5% of single duct discharges are caused by intraduct cancers. The presence of blood in the discharge does not aid the differentiation of malignant from benign causes; cytology of the discharge may be useful. Until recently therefore single duct discharge was treated in our centre by microdochectomy (excision of the involved duct): the histological results of 178 cases treated by this method are shown in table 10.2. A re-evaluation of these cases showed that in the 11 cases of intraduct carcinoma found which had been sent for mammography preoperatively, nine showed changes suspicious of carcinoma. We have therefore changed our management: the sequence now is to separate multiple and single duct discharges, examine and

**Table 10.2**   Histopathology of 179 cases undergoing
microdochectomy for single duct nipple discharge

| Histopathological diagnosis | Number of patients |
| --- | --- |
| Ductal carcinoma *in situ* | 12 |
| Intraduct papilloma | 77 |
| Other benign breast disease | 80 |
| No specific abnormality | 1 |

then mammogram the latter. If neither of these shows an abnormality the patient is seen again in one year: if the discharge persists a further mammogram is taken, and if again normal she is not followed up further. If we had used this management in the 178 cases we would have advised microdochectomy in only 30. If a patient wishes to be rid of the discharge despite our reassurance, then we accede to her request.

## Microdochectomy

This operation may be carried out under local anaesthetic although many patients prefer general anaesthesia day case surgery. On the day of admission the patient is examined to ensure that discharge can still be expressed and this is again checked in the anaesthetic room.

The surgeon may prefer to wear a magnifying hood. The duct is identified and a lacrymal probe is placed in it and advanced as far as it will easily pass (usually about 3 cm). A silk suture is then placed at the nipple and the probe tied in firmly. The skin over the probe is infiltrated with 1 in 80 000 adrenaline solution and an incision made over the length of the probe. The skin edges are each held back with a suture (Fig. 10.5).

The duct is freed along its length as far as possible – multiple divisions finally making this difficult. If discharge is coming from the divisions then each of these is further followed for 1–2 cm as they are divided. The duct may lead to a lesion: a localised area of cystic disease or a small solid carcinoma *in situ*. Otherwise once the duct has been freed it is opened, and a papilloma may be found (Fig. 10.6). The skin is closed with 4.0 polypropylene sutures after careful haemostasis, leaving a suction drain if a solid area was excised.

## Nipple eczema

Eczema of the nipple, or nipple and areola, in the absence of a palpable lump is likely to be caused by Paget's disease. A history that the nipple has healed on occasions may be obtained, as temporary healing may occur.

The diagnosis is simple. In the clinic the nipple is anaesthetised with local anaesthetic containing adrenaline. A sliver biopsy specimen is taken with a No. 11 scalpel blade used without a handle, and one small stitch is inserted. Histology shows the typical changes: as an intraduct carcinoma further discussion of Paget's disease is beyond the scope of this book.

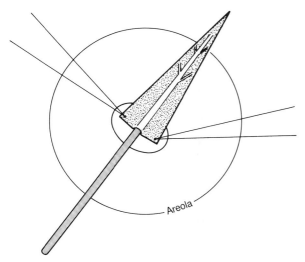

**Fig 10.5**   The operation of microdochectomy.

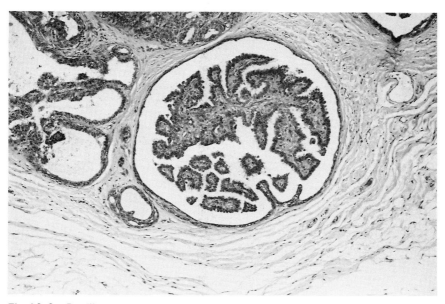

**Fig 10.6**   Papilloma in a large duct.

## Mamillary fistula and periareola abscess

Duct ectasia – dilated ducts under the nipple with inspissated secretions, periductal fibrosis, and inflammation – is a common condition in women in the 40–60 age group. This has been shown by incidental histology of biopsies or microdochectomies and is associated with dilated ducts which may be seen on mammograms (Fig. 10.7).

The static secretion within these ducts is prone to infection by anaerobes. Once infection is present then it is difficult to clear, as in similar conditions with static material, like bronchiectasis. The infection results in small abscesses presenting at the edge of the areola. These are frequently recurrent. This condition predisposes to mamillary fistula: the infected duct forms an abscess which discharges through the skin leaving a fistula (Fig. 10.8). There may be a residual lump after such discharge or a low grade, chronic infection.

At first presentation in the acute phase the abscess is incised and if possible the fistula found. A probe is passed up the duct through the nipple and an incision made up to the nipple; the wound is then left to granulate.

On recurrence the best operation is to excise the central ducts (Hadfield's procedure, mammodochectomy). This operation can also be used for a multiple duct discharge for which the patient wishes treatment.

### Excision of the central ducts

The lower edge of the areola is carefully marked with a pen and an accurate cut made around the lower circumference. Nipple and areola are raised from

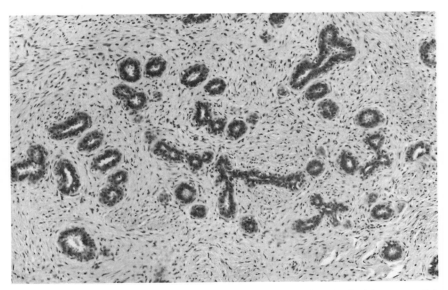

**Fig 10.7**   Mammogram showing dilated ducts under the nipple (duct ectasia).

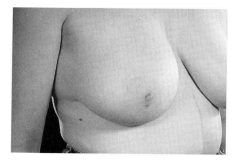

**Fig 10.8**  Mamilary fistula.

the breast by a horizontal scalpel cut with a No. 15 blade, cutting a minimum thickness of around 5 mm of tissue subcutaneously. A 23 blade then cuts straight down into the breast tissue (Fig. 10.9) in a circle directly under the areola edge to a depth of 2 cms. The subareolar block of tissue is excised. The subcutaneous dissection around the areola is extended for about 1–2 cm, and then the deep tissue is apposed with an absorbable suture and the skin resutured with 4.0 polypropylene over a suction drain.

## Breast abscess: haematoma and fat necrosis

Breast abscess in relation to mamillary fistula has been discussed above. An acute abscess occurring anywhere within the breast is relatively common in pregnancy and is dealt with by incision when 'ripe' for doing so. Although the incision must be generous enough to let out the pus it does not have to be large and it can be placed cosmetically: the incision is closed around a Latex drain. There is no reason for through and through incisions giving dependent drainage as have sometimes been advocated. The Latex drain is removed as soon as pus is no longer draining.

Breast abscess outside the puerperium is usually straightforward, but may rarely be associated with malignancy: there is more likely to be confusion when an abscess is not well defined, giving an oedematous breast with general inflammation which may resemble an inflammatory carcinoma widely spread through the breast. An abscess outside the puerperium is

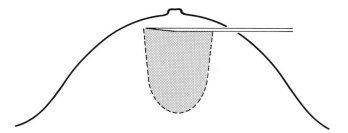

**Fig 10.9**   The operation of excision of the central breast ducts.

incised on the usual merits but a biopsy of the wall should be taken; if it has presented early then antibiotics may abort the abscess. If this course is taken a Trucut biopsy is carried out once the acute inflammation has settled to ensure that only inflammatory tissue is seen. The lump must then resolve completely over the next two months both clinically and on mammography carried out four weeks later. If a lesion is still present clinically or mammographically, surgical excision is advisable.

Traumatic haemotoma/fat necrosis often presents as a breast lump in women in their seventies. To accept this as a possible diagnosis there must be a clear history of trauma and of an obvious bruise, as patients not infrequently rationalise a cancerous lump to be due to some past trauma. If such a clear history is given then a Trucut biopsy is taken: as long as this shows only fat necrosis the lump is watched for complete resolution clinically and later mammographically. Failure to resolve within two months indicates the need for excision biopsy.

## Conclusion

The breast is an important structure to a woman's psychology for all the reasons usually quoted. Scarring the breast and discomfort from postoperative haematomas are to be avoided if possible. On the other hand, operation to exclude malignant disease may be the safe course. Structured evaluation and the use of aspiration cytology reduce the need for such surgery but clear protocols must be drawn up and adhered to. Operation on the breast is simple but requires care to achieve a good cosmetic result and to avoid complications.

# 11

# Plastic surgery techniques for non-malignant breast disease

JOHN AE HOBBY

Reconstructive surgery for benign disease of the breast involves treating patients with small breasts by augmentation mammaplasty, large breasts by breast reduction, and sagging breasts by mastopexy. Breast asymmetry may be treated by augmentation or reduction mammaplasty. Breast reconstruction is used to treat patients with congenital aplasia of the breast and after subcutaneous mastectomy[1] or damage to the breast by trauma.

Scars on the breast for some of the above procedures are extensive and may, in white skinned patients, result in postoperative hypertrophic scars which take up to two years or more to settle. Scars in black or brown skinned patients may result in keloid formation, an even more difficult problem to deal with. Careful placement of scars is essential to ensure satisfactory results, and all patients should have preoperative marking of proposed incision sites, made while they are standing, with an indelible marker pen. At operation the patient is placed supine with elbows slightly flexed and hands flat under the flanks. All pressure points should be protected by foam cushions. The patient should be placed in the sitting position between 45° and 60° from the horizontal. This results in some ptosis of the breasts and helps to obtain a satisfactory aesthetic result.

## Mammary augmentation

Social pressures and modern advertising techniques place considerable psychological stress on women with small breasts. Sometimes this leads to feelings of inadequacy in these women who seek to solve their emotional problems by undergoing breast augmentation. The indications for augmentation mammaplasty may be grouped under the following headings: (a) developmental hypoplasia, (b) idiopathic involution of breast tissue following pregnancy, (c) sudden weight loss in small breasted women, and (d) mammary assymetry.

Not all patients seeking augmentation after idiopathic involution following pregnancy have small breasts. Some patients seek correction of drooping of the breasts, and with it an apparent loss of tissue above the nipples. Their request is that the breasts be 'filled out'. These patients present a difficult problem which may be dealt with by augmentation, by mastopexy, or a combination of these procedures. Contra-indications to mammary augmentation are: (a) recent breast abscess, (b) diffuse cystic mastitis, (c) marked breast ptosis, (d) a breast tumour, or (e) severe psychosexual problems.

Historically the percutaneous injection of paraffin and silicone preparations have been used to enlarge breast size, but these methods are now condemned. Local flaps of dermis fat, and free dermis fat grafts from areas such as the buttock have been used, but these methods have been superseded by the use of prosthetic material. In the 1950s, polyvinyl sponge was used but this material underwent a change after implantation for long periods, and produced sarcomas in rats.[2] Sponge implants have now been replaced by silicone bag implants. The most commonly used prosthetic implant for breast augmentation is a derivative of that first described by Cronin and Gerow.[3] It consists of a Silastic envelope filled with silicone gel. No association has been demonstrated between breast carcinoma and silicone breast prostheses.

Inflatable prostheses consisting of a silicone bag filled with Dextran or isotonic saline have been described.[4] These prostheses can be introduced via small circumareolar incisions, but are prone to rupture and deflation. Polyurethane coated breast implants have the major advantage of lack of capsule formation and contraction around the implant, which is important complication of silicone implants.[5, 6]

General anaesthesia is used for the operation and local infiltration of the incision with 1% lignocaine containing 1 in 80 000 adrenaline reduces bleeding. All powder should be washed from surgical gloves, or powder free gloves used, in order to prevent powder granuloma which may contribute to later capsular contraction. A submammary transverse incision above the inframammary fold 5 cm in length is made. In an average patient, the medial extremity of the incision is 7 cm from the midline. The advantage of an incision above the inframammary groove is that the base of the breast can be approached in an oblique subcutaneous plane, so that when closing the wound a cushion of breast tissue buttresses the implant from the skin wound (Fig. 11.1(a) and (b) ). Alternatively, an axillary approach posterior to the anterior axillary fold can be used, but it is necessary to use a special long blunt dissector to reach the inferior margin of the breast.

## Submammary augmentation

The submammary pocket is created when one reaches the fascia covering pectoralis major at the inferior margin of the breast. Initially the dissection commences between the muscle fascia and the posterior capsule of the breast with blunt curved scissors. It is then possible to introduce the index finger into an easily dissectable, virtually bloodless tissue plane. The plane is

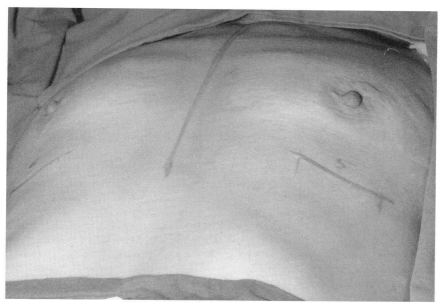

**Fig 11.1a**   Incision marks before augmentation.

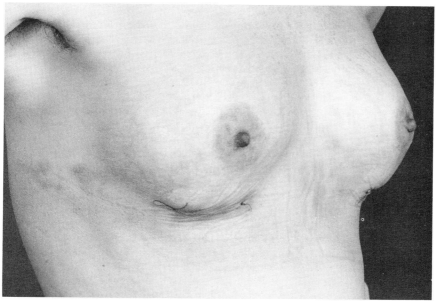

**Fig 11.1b**   Ten days after augmentation.

developed with a sweeping motion of the index finger. A circular base of approximately 14 cm is created in the average patient. It is necessary to divide fibrous attachments between the skin and costal cartilages inferiomedially. Failure to free these attachments may result in a prosthesis being placed too laterally. At this stage, haemostasis should be secured. Commonly one has to coagulate perforating arteries, usually two, which emanate from the lower medial origin of pectoralis major.

## Subpectoral augmentation

To reduce the rate of post augmentation capsular contraction silicone prostheses can be placed in the submuscular plane. The incision and approach are as already described, but the subglandular dissection is limited to exposing the lower fibres of pectoralis major. At this stage a muscle splitting incision is performed, exposing the underlying ribs. A submuscular plane is then developed between pectoralis major above, rectus abdominis below, and serratus anterior laterally. Care must be taken not to develop the subpectoral plane too far superiorly, as the prosthesis will sit too high and give an unsatisfactory result. The wound is closed in layers with absorbable sutures and finally the skin is closed with intradermal polypropylene (Prolene) sutures, which are removed two weeks following surgery. At the end of the procedure a compression bodice is applied to the chest and worn for a period of six weeks following surgery. This garment limits the likelihood of postoperative haematoma and helps to control the position of the prostheses postoperatively.

Early complications are uncommon, although haematoma formation and infection are possible. Either of these complications may require reoperation to control bleeding or remove the foreign body (prosthesis) to control infection. Wound breakdown is rare but if this does occur the patient should be warned that loss of the prosthesis is likely.

Since their introduction in the early 1960s, silicone prostheses have proved to be safe and in many cases soft and mobile. They are not without complications, however, and physical complications include rupture of the prosthesis, which may be spontaneous or traumatic. New high performance Silastic is now used for the silicone bag envelope in the latest generation of implants, and spontaneous rupture of these prostheses is uncommon. The main complication with silicone prostheses is the physiological one of capsular contraction. All prostheses are encapsulated by the host. Why capsular contraction occurs is a complex problem and the cause is unknown. Capsular contraction is often unilateral which mitigates against circulating humoral or systemic factors. Silicone droplets have been considered, but capsular contraction also occurs around saline filled prostheses. The infection theory implicates subclinical infection with *Staphylococcus epidermidis*,[7] a bacterium found on skin and in nipple secretions. The explanation of how this subclinical infection leads to capsular contraction has yet to be elucidated.

Of the non-infectious causes, hereditary disposition, granuloma from glove powder, and haematoma have been suggested. Laboratory evidence implicates myofibroblast cells associated with haematoma formation. Greater numbers of myofibroblasts are present in contracted capsules than in non-contracted capsules. Myofibroblast density peaks, and then declines, after the active contraction phase of wound healing. Capsular contraction is not necessarily an early phenomenon, and I have seen it for the first time in a patient two years following mammary augmentation. Late capsular contraction occurs after the myofibroblast population has declined, and is not likely to be the explanation in these cases. Clinical capsular contraction is preceded by pain in the affected breast in most patients; the breast then becomes firm and, later, hard to palpation. Breast shape becomes distorted and the prosthesis rides up and the nipple down.

Scheflan[8] in a review of 1000 patients after breast augmentation found a detectable firmness rate of 60%. This is my experience and patients should be made aware that some degree of firmness in one or both of their augmented breasts is likely in one out of every two cases. This figure is true for subglandular augmentation but can be reduced to one in five patients by using the submuscular method. Capsular contraction has been classified by Baker *et al.*[9]

- Grade I: The augmented breast feels as soft as the unoperated one.
- Grade II: The breast is less soft: the implant can be palpated, but is not visible.
- Grade III: The breast is more firm; the implant can be palpated easily, and it (or distortion from it) can be seen.
- Grade IV: The breast is hard, tender, painful and cold. Distortion is often marked.

Baker *et al* described the closed compression technique for rupturing a contracted capsule around a breast implant. In this technique the surgeon clasps his hands together, interlocking the fingers. The firm breast capsule is clasped by the heels of the hands and pressure applied to tear the capsule. This manoeuvre is uncomfortable and sometimes painful for the patient. It is normally performed in the outpatient clinic, but sometimes patients request a short general anaesthetic. Closed capsulotomy may be repeated, and provided the patient presents with a Grade II or Grade III contracture, capsular contraction is normally easily accomplished. Grade IV contractures are more difficult to treat, and sometimes open capsulotomy is necessary for correction. Rarely patients request removal of their prostheses. Closed capsulotomy may be complicated by haematoma, which should be managed conservatively and normally settles. Excessive force may lead to rupture of the prosthesis with subsequent distortion of shape as the gel leaks from the bag; in these cases reoperation is necessary.

Although submuscular placement of the prostheses lowers the incidence of clinically detectable capsular contraction, it does not eliminate it. Closed capsulotomy is more difficult to achieve when the prosthesis is in the submuscular position. Additionally, the strong contraction of pectoralis major sometimes distorts the breast shape along the lateral border of the muscle, and patients should be warned of this. When a large prosthesis is used in a small patient, I have seen the breast ride up over the prosthesis on strong contraction of pectoralis major. This gives an unpleasant shape to the breast and is best treated by placing the prosthesis in the subglandular position. The choice of subglandular or submuscular augmentation is not always a clear cut one. I use the submuscular method for extremely small breasted patients, and use a prosthesis no greater than 210 ml capacity. Where breast volume is greater, prostheses up to and in excess of 300 ml may be used in the subglandular position.

Polyurethane coated breast prostheses may in time supersede present prostheses. The major advantage claimed for these prostheses is the lack of capsule formation around them, and absence of postaugmentation capsular contraction. There is, however, an incomplete understanding of the fate of polyurethane when implanted in humans, and these implants have not yet been generally accepted. Some reports of complications using these implants are beginning to appear.[10, 11] Mammary augmentation takes place behind the breast tissue, therefore, breast function is undisturbed and subsequent breast masses should not be concealed. In raising the breast from the underlying pectoralis major, the sensory nerve supply to the nipple which comes through the lateral border of the muscle is sometimes stretched. This can lead to a decrease in sensation of the nipple.

## Breast asymmetry

Minor forms of breast asymmetry can be corrected with simple subglandular silicone augmentation (Fig. 11.2(a) and (b) ). In this type of case, capsular contraction is less common. This may be related to the fact that one is augmenting a breast of ample proportion and there is a large amount of breast tissue covering the implant. Large degrees of breast inequality may best be managed using the technique of tissue expansion which is described later.

## Reduction mammaplasty and mastopexy

Heavy pendulous breasts can be both a physical and mental handicap. In a young patient with pubertal hypertrophy they may be a social embarrassment and interfere with sporting activities. In the older patient the complaints are more often pain in the drooping breasts and associated pain in the back and neck. Kyphosis and arthritis of the cervical spine may develop as a consequence of poor posture associated with large breasts.[12] Bra straps often cut into the shoulders, producing obvious indentation of the skin. In warm weather, intertrigo between and beneath the breasts is a common complaint. Breast hypertrophy in older patients is often associated with chronic mastitis, and breast reduction may help to decrease pain by reducing the amount of breast tissue and the gravitational drag on the breasts.

Breast asymmetry can be corrected by unilateral breast reduction. In the young patient, unilateral augmentation is normally the best procedure because of the scarring involved with breast reduction. In the older patient, however, often in association with breast reconstruction following

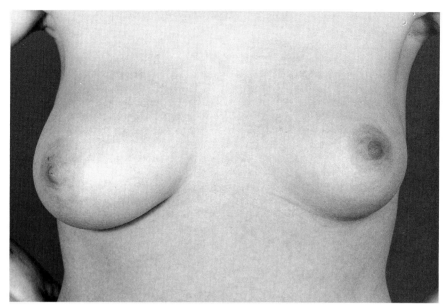

**Fig 11.2a**   Before augmentation of the left breast.

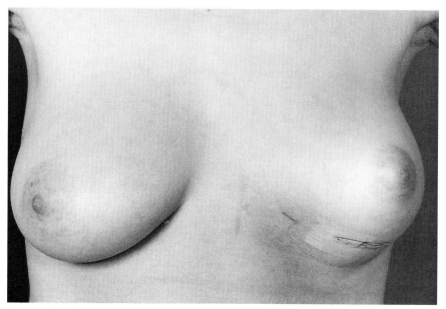

**Fig 11.2b**   Ten days after augmentation.

mastectomy, unilateral breast reduction or mastopexy may be performed to achieve breast symmetry.

Historically, early breast reduction techniques involved free transfer of the nipple/areola complex as a full thickness graft.[13, 14] Free nipple transfer is associated with loss of function as far as lactation is concerned and, more importantly, loss of nipple sensation. In an attempt to overcome these problems various pedicle techniques have been described, where the nipple remains attached either to a dermal pedicle or to a parenchymal one. The lateral pedicle technique of Strömbeck[15, 16] was the first of these, followed by the vertical pedicles described by McKissock.[17] Variations on the vertical pedicle technique involve a single superior pedicle[18] and a single inferior pedicle.[19]

In a series of 300 cases using the inferior pedicle technique[20] the most common complication was minor suture line necrosis along the inframammary incision. There were no cases of necrosis or sensory loss of the nipple/areolar complex. The inferior pedicle technique is safe with a low complication rate, and can be used for extremely large breasts. The nipple heights can be raised by up to 20 cm and one rarely needs to use the free nipple transfer technique. The breasts and local lymph nodes must be carefully examined prior to surgery, and if necessary mammograms performed to exclude breast disease.

Preoperative marking of the breasts must be made with the patient standing (Fig. 11.3(a) ). Initially, the suprasternal notch should be marked and the midclavicular point identified. A line is then drawn from this point to the nipple. The line is then projected further to the inframammary fold

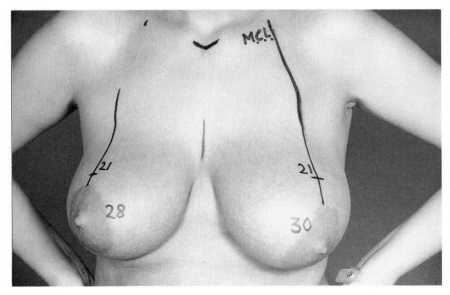

**Fig 11.3a**   Preoperative markings for reduction mammaplasty.

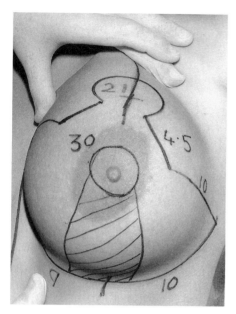

**Fig 11.3b** Completed markings.

(Fig. 11.3(b) ). The distance from the suprasternal notch to the nipple is then measured. It is common for the height of the nipples to vary between 1 and 2 cm from each other. The new height for the nipple is then marked on the midclavicular line. This position should be over the inframammary crease, and can be judged by using the examining thumb and index finger in the maximum pinch position; this height is normally between 20 and 22 cm from the suprasternal notch. Great care must be taken not to place the nipples too high, or they will ride up above a covering bra. This is distressing to the patient, and an extremely difficult problem to correct. At this stage a line just above the inframammary crease is marked, the approximate centre of which has already been marked as an extension of the midclavicular line. Alternatively, this line can be marked at the time of surgery. After preparing and draping the patient further incision lines are marked (Fig. 11.3(c) ). A circular area around the nipple 4 cm in diameter is marked. A keyhole pattern is then drawn at the new nipple height.[21] The vertical limbs of the keyhole pattern are made 4.5 cm long. The inferior extremities of the lines are then joined to the extremities of the inframammary marking, both medially and laterally. The inferior pedicle is then marked. Care must be taken not to encroach on the midline over the manubrium, as scars placed in this position are a disaster. They will become hypertrophic and lead to web contracture which is virtually impossible to correct.

The operation commences with the cutting of the inferior pedicle (Fig.11.3(d) ). I routinely leave a dermal pedicle but this is not essential, and the nipple may be attached to a parenchymal pedicle only.[20] Breast tissue is then excised down to the fascia of pectoralis major along the previously

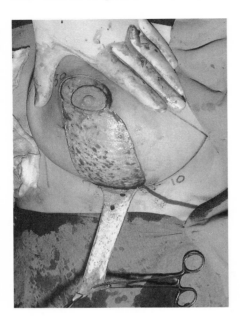

**Fig 11.3c**  The de-epithelialised inferior pedicle.

marked incision lines. No undermining of the breast flaps is necessary. A thin covering of breast tissue is left over the lateral muscle in order to preserve the nerve supply to the nipple. It is possible using buried absorbable 2/0 sutures to join the inferior margins of the keyhole incision with the extension of the midclavicular line on the inframammary incision (Fig. 11.3(e) and (f)). Further 2/0 absorbable deep sutures are used to approximate the wound edges, and finally a 3/0 intradermal polypropylene suture completes wound closure. Around the areola a 4/0 absorbable suture is used to close areola to skin (Fig. 11.3(g)). Support for the breasts using an adequate bra for three or four months following surgery aids early resolution of scars and minimises scar stretching.

## Mastopexy

Bilateral mastopexy is requested for drooping breasts where the patient is happy with the breast volumes. The preoperative marking of the patient is the same as in breast reduction, excluding only the marking of the inferior pedicle. No breast tissue is removed and wide undermining of the uppper medial and lateral skin flaps from the underlying breast parenchyma is necessary. Care must be taken not to devitalize the skin flaps, and meticulous haemostasis is essential. The pre-operative and six month post-operative result of such a procedure is shown in Fig. 11.4(a) and (b). The early three week scarring after breast reduction Fig. 11.3(f) and (g)) is contrasted with the six month result after mastopexy (Fig. 11.4(b)). With time the breast shape improves and scars fade well, provided that adequate post-operative support is maintained.

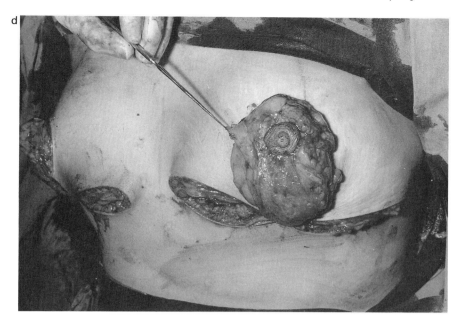

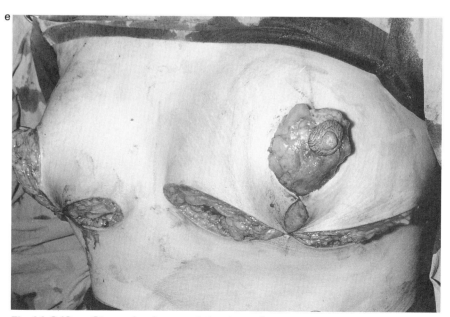

**Fig 11.3d&e**   Stages in closure of the wound.

f

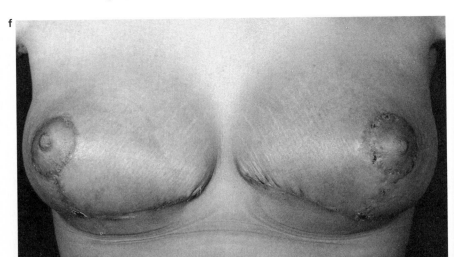

g

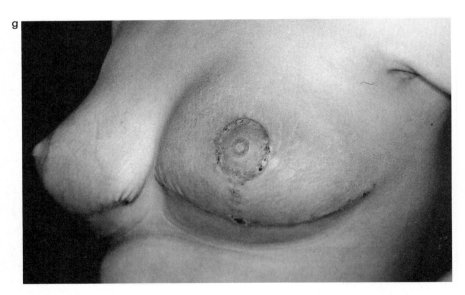

**Fig 11.3f&g**   Scars three weeks after bilateral reduction mammoplasty.

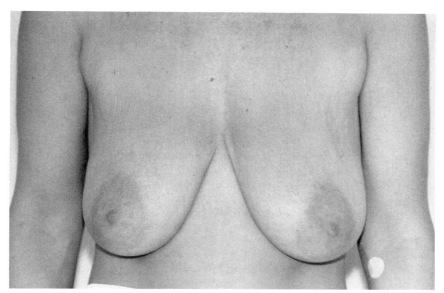

**Fig 11.4a**  Before bilateral mastopexy.

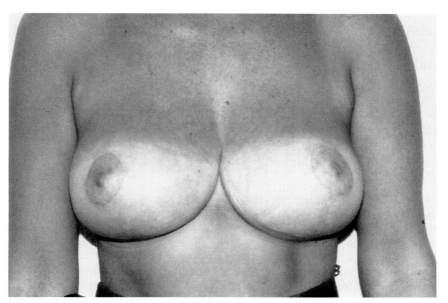

**Fig 11.4b**  Six months after bilateral mastopexy.

Unilateral mastopexy is required in the young patient after removal of a giant benign juvenile fibroadenoma. Such a case is shown in Fig. 11.5(a) and (b). These cases are often more complex as is highlighted in this young girl whose nipple/areola complex was displaced inferiorly and laterally.

## Complications of reduction mammoplasty and mastopexy

Breast reduction and mastopexy using the inferior pedicle technique are remarkably free of early and late complications. Immediate problems are related to haematoma formation, which is minimised by adequate haemostasis at the time of surgery and postoperative drainage for two days. Minor disruption of the suture line is uncommon, and when it occurs is related to the junction of the vertical midline breast scar where it meets the inframammary incision. This problem invariably settles with local conservative management. Fat necrosis in fat patients may be a troublesome problem, and lead to persistent sinus drainage. I have not seen this problem with the inferior pedicle technique. Hypertrophic scar formation may be a problem, but normally settles if adequate time is allowed to elapse, and good breast support is maintained. Troublesome pain and irritation in scars is occasionally helped by applying Silastic gel sheeting to the wounds. Local steroid injections should be avoided, as pronounced thinning and stretching of the scars will result. Recurrence of deformity following reduction and mastopexy can occur[22] and patients should be warned of this. Fluctuations in weight, ageing, and pregnancy can compromise an initially satisfactory result.

## Subcutaneous mastectomy

Subcutaneous mastectomy has been advocated for benign breast disease.[1] The arguments as to the correctness of subcutaneous mastectomy for prophylaxis against carcinoma are controversial and outside the scope of this chapter. Requests for subcutaneous mastectomy are made, however, and patients may be divided into the following groups: (a) fibrocystic disease, (b) intractable mastalgia, (c) refractory suppurative mastitis, and silicone granuloma.

Subcutaneous mastectomy fails to remove all breast tissue. A small button of ductal and breast tissue is left under the nipple/areola complex, and a remnant of breast may be left in the axillary tail of the breast.[23] The early results of subcutaneous mastectomy and placement of the silicone prosthesis beneath the skin flaps lead to unacceptably high complication rates. Secondary reconstruction, normally three months later, reduces the early complication rate but not the late major complication of capsular contraction. The case for immediate submuscular reconstruction has been made by Woods *et al.*[24] Long term follow up is necessary in these patients in order fully to assess the complications. Slade,[25] in a report of the results of 88 patients, found an overall surgical complication rate of 25%. The complications in order of frequency were flap necrosis, nipple loss, haematoma requiring surgery or aspiration, infection, and implant extrusion. Immediate

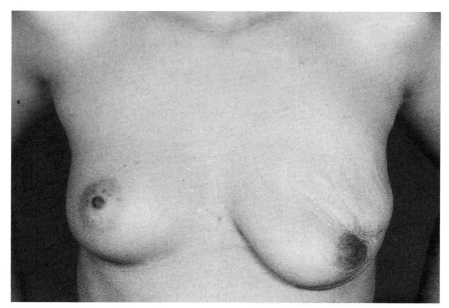

**Fig 11.5a** Before left mastopexy.

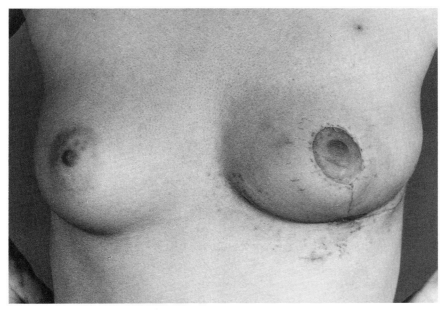

**Fig 11.5b** After left mastopexy.

reconstruction had the highest complication rate (39%), and all the implant extrusions occurred in this group. Delayed reconstruction had a complication rate of 16%. The major long term problem in these cases is similar to that of mammary augmentation, namely, capsular contraction. Subcutaneous placement of the prostheses resulted in a 100% rate of capsular contraction, whereas subpectoral placement of the prostheses resulted in a capsular contraction rate of 50%.

Radovan (Radovan C. Adjacent flap development using expandable Silastic implants. Presented at American Society of Plastic and Reconstructive Surgery, Surgical Forum, Boston, 1976)[26] and Austad and Rose[27] evolved the technology for the safe expansion of soft tissues. The technique of tissue expansion can be used in reconstruction after subcutaneous mastectomy; the surgical method and type of reconstruction needs to be tailored to the individual patient. Where immediate reconstruction is contemplated the prosthesis must be placed in the submuscular plane. If the pectoralis fascia is removed with the subcutaneous mastectomy specimen, there is a limit to the size of silicone prosthesis which can be accommodated in the submuscular space. The prosthesis must not be greater than 300 ml or it will rupture from the submuscular plane along the lateral border of pectoralis major. In women with large breasts this will involve reduction of skin at the time of mastectomy. This can be achieved using the mastopexy method already described (leaving the nipple attached to a dermal pedicle), but it may result in total nipple/areolar loss.

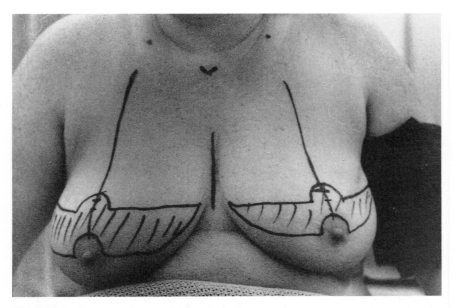

**Fig 11.6a**  Preoperative markings for subcutaneous mastectomy, transverse approach.

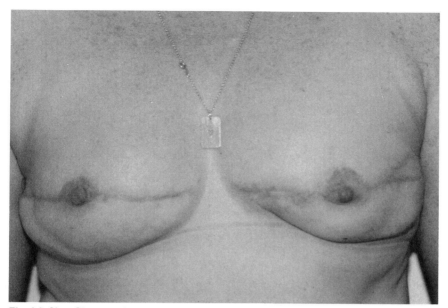

**Fig 11.6b**   Six months after bilateral subcutaneous mastectomy.

A better approach is to use a transverse incision and upper skin flaps which can either be de-epithelialised and used as a buttress to the upper skin flap, or discarded. This technique provides good exposure to perform an adequate mastectomy with total removal of the gland, axillary tail, and axillary glands if necessary (Fig. 11.6(a) and (b) ). This technique is particularly useful in cases of silicone granuloma (Fig. 11.7). In these rare cases reconstruction should be undertaken at a second stage by submuscular augmentation or tissue expansion.

The need to excise skin at the time of subcutaneous mastectomy can be reduced by using tissue expansion. At the time of mastectomy, or as a delayed procedure, a tissue expander can be introduced into a submuscular pocket and the inflation valve sited in the axilla or over the opposite costal cartilages (Fig. 11.8(a),(b) and (c) ). At the time of surgery 150–200 ml of normal saline can be introduced into the expander using several 20 ml syringes on a 23 gauge needle. Weekly during the postoperative period, further saline can be introduced until over expansion of the breast skin is obtained. In a small breast a 500 ml expander will suffice, but larger breasts will need a 1000 ml tissue expander. When the required expansion has been obtained the expander can be removed and replaced with a permanent silicone implant. The exact size of the implant needed is equivalent to the volume of saline required to achieve breast symmetry (Fig. 11.8). In this case, right subcutaneous mastectomy and reconstruction were performed following left mastectomy for lobular carcinoma. The left breast has been

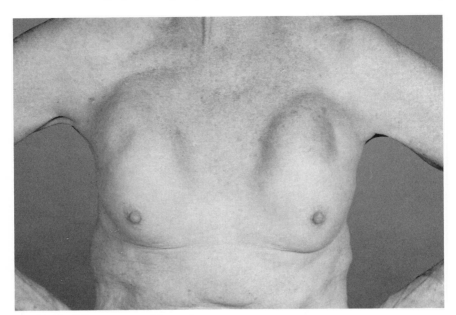

**Fig 11.7**   Siliconomas of breast.

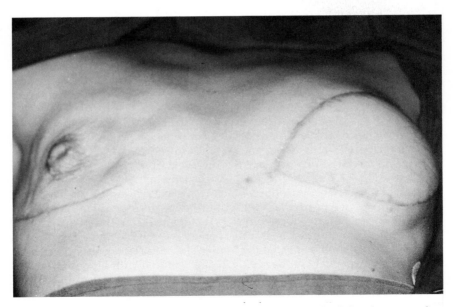

**Fig 11.8a** Before secondary tissue expansion of right breast after subcutaneous mastectomy.

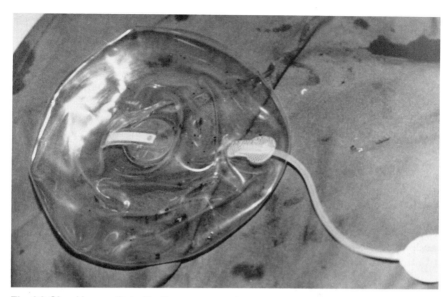

**Fig 11.8b**   Heyer–Schulte tissue expander.

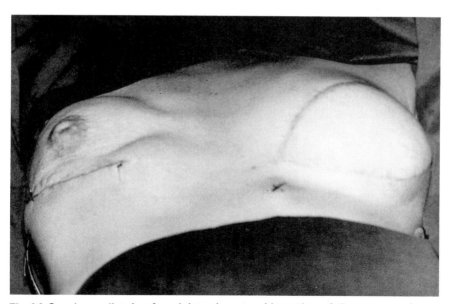

**Fig 11.8c**   Immediately after right subpectoral insertion of tissue expander.

reconstructed using a latissimus dorsi flap and awaits later nipple areolar reconstruction.[28, 29, 30]

## Breast reconstruction

Total replacement of the breast is required in patients with Poland's syndrome.[31] In this anomaly there is total absence of breast tissue associated with a congenital abnormality of the ipsilateral upper limb. A young girl with transverse arrest of development in her right midforearm is shown in Fig. 11.9(a) and (b), associated with absence of her right breast and pectoralis major muscle. This deformity can be corrected in a single stage procedure by transposing latissimus dorsi to the anterior chest wall, and then augmentating it with a silicone prosthesis.[32] The patient is placed on her side on the operating table and the procedure performed by an approach along the posterior axillary line. The latissimus dorsi flap can be raised as an island, leaving the supplying thoracodorsal neurovascular bundle intact. The tendinous insertion of the muscle is divided from the humerus and is inserted into the anterior capsule of the shoulder to create an anterior axillary line. A suitable silicone prosthesis is then inserted under the muscle which is secured around it. Broad spectrum peroperative antibiotics are administered, and vacuum drains should be left *in situ* in the anterior and posterior wounds for four days to prevent postoperative haematoma formation.

The breast may need to be reconstructed after injury. A major flame burn as a child resulted in extensive damage to the left chest, abdomen and

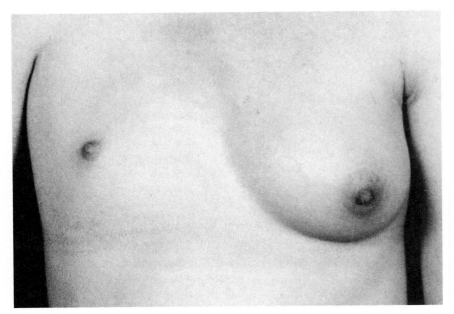

**Fig 11.9a**   Poland's syndrome (right breast) before operation.

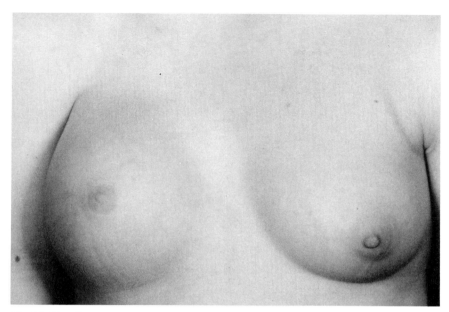

**Fig 11.9b**  Result after reconstruction.

posterior thorax in the patient shown (Fig. 11.10(a) and (b) ). A latissimus dorsi myocutaneous flap reconstruction was ruled out by the extent of the burn, and tissue expansion under burn scar is likely to produce a poor result. New tissue to reconstruct her left breast was introduced using a contralateral transverse rectus abdominis flap.[33, 34] In this procedure a transverse abdominal skin and subcutaneous fat flap was raised on the contralateral rectus abdominis. The supplying vascular bundle to this flap is via the deep superior epigastric vessels which run on the under surface of the rectus. A diamond shaped skin flap can be taken from the umbilicus above to the mons pubis below. Laterally the flap can extend from the anterior iliac spine on the side containing the vascular trunk to two thirds of the way from the midline to the anterior iliac spine on the opposite side. The upper abdominal skin is then undermined and brought down to meet the lower incision with resiting of the umbilicus. The transverse rectus abdominis flap is technically more difficult to perform than the latissimus dorsi flap, and great care must be exercised not to occlude the supplying vascular pedicle when transposing the muscle.

A similar technique was used to correct radionecrosis of the chest in a lady 20 years after radiotherapy for carcinoma of the left breast (Fig. 11.11(a) and (b) ). Initially the area of radionecrosis on the anterior and lateral chest walls was excised, and replaced with an ipsilateral transverse rectus abdominis flap. Six months later the left breast was augmented with a 500 ml silicone prosthesis to obtain symmetry.

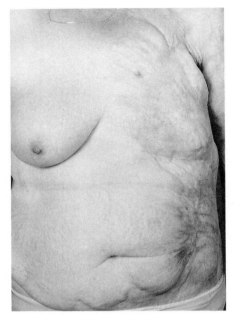

**Fig 11.10a**   Burn to left breast

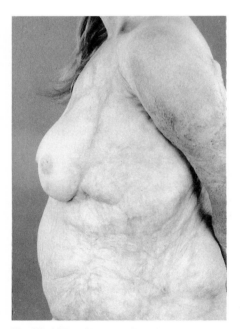

**Fig 11.10b**   Six months after reconstruction. The nipple was reconstructed by the tattooing technique.

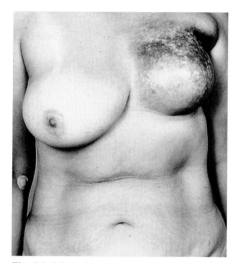

**Fig 11.11a** Radionecrosis of the left breast.

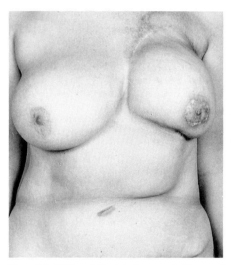

**Fig 11.11b** After augmentation of the left breast and nipple/areola reconstruction.

## Nipple/areola reconstruction

The nipple is best replaced by sharing the opposite 2–3 mm of nipple as a free graft. The areola can be reconstructed using a full thickness skin graft taken from the non-hair bearing groin skin. The tissues may be transplanted as free grafts onto a de-epethialised base as shown in Fig. 11.1. If use of the opposite nipple is inappropriate a nipple can be reconstructed using a subcutaneous cone of tisue;[35] alternatively, labia minora can be used.[36] Full thickness grafts to reconstruct the areola can sometimes be followed by hypopigmentation of these grafts. This can be corrected by tattooing, which in some cases can recreate the appearance of an areola without the need for grafting.

## References

1. Freeman BS. Subcutaneous mastectomy for benign breast lesions with immediate or delayed prosthetic replacement. *Plast Reconstr Surg* 1962; **30**: 676–682.
2. Dukes CE, Mitchley MI. Polyvinyl sponge implants. *Br J Plast Surg* 1962; **15**: 225.
3. Cronin TD, Gerow F. Augmentation mammaplasty: a new 'natural feel' prosthesis. In: *Transactions Third International Plastic Surgery*. Amsterdam, Excerpta Medica, 1964, pp. 41–49.
4. Arion HG. Retromammary prosthesis. Comptes Rendus Societe Français Gynecologie 1965; **5**: 427–431.
5. Ashley FL. A new type of breast prosthesis – preliminary report. *Plast Reconstr Surg* 1970; **45**: 421–424.
6. Herman S. The meme implant. *Plast Reconstr Surg* 1984; **73**: 411–414.
7. Burkhardt CR, Fried M, Schnur PL, Tofield JJ. Capsule infection and intra luminal antibiotic. *Plast Reconstr Surg* 1981; **68**: 43–49.
8. Scheflan M, Kalisman M. Complications of breast reconstruction. *Clin Plast Surg* 1984; **2**: 343–50.
9. Baker JC, Bartels KJ, Douglas WM. Closed compression technique for rupturing a contracted capsule around a breast implant. *Plast Reconstr Surg* 1976; **58**: 137–139.
10. Jabaley ME, Das SK. Late breast pain following reconstruction with polyurethane covered implants. *Plast Reconstr Surg* 1986; **78**: 390–95.
11. Okunski WJ, Chowdary RP. Infected meme implants: salvage reconstruction with latissimus dorsi myocutaneous flaps and silicone implants. *Aesthetic Plast Surg* 1987; **2**: 49–51.
12. Conway H. Mammaplasty: analysis of 110 consecutive cases with end results. *Plast Reconstr Surg* 1952; **10**: 303–315.
13. Thorek M. Possibilities in the reconstruction of the human form. *NY Med J Rec* 1922; **116**: 572.
14. Thorek M. Plastic Reconstruction of the breast and free transplantation of the nipple. *Journal of the International College of Surgeons* 1946; **9**: 194–197.
15. Strömbeck JG. Mammaplasty: report of a new technique based on the two-pedicle procedure. *Br J Plast Surg* 1960 **13**: 79–90.
16. Strömbeck JG. Reduction mammaplasty. In: Grabb W, Smith JW. (Eds) *Plastic Surgery. A Concise Guide to Clinical Practise*. Boston, Little, Brown and Company, 1968, pp. 821–35.
17  McKissock PK. Reduction mammaplasty with a vertical dermal flap. *Plast Reconstr Surg* 1972; **49**: 245–52.

18. Wiener DL, Adrien EA, Aiache E, *et al*. A single dermal pedicle for nipple transposition in subcutaneous mastectomy, reduction mammaplasty, or mastopexy. *Plast Reconstr Surg* 1973; **51**: 115–120.
19. Courtiss EH, Goldwyn RM. Reduction mammoplasty by the inferior pedicle technique: an alternative to full nipple and areola grafting for severe macromastia or extreme ptosis. *Plastic Reconstr Surg* 1977; **59**: 400–07.
20. Bolger WE, Seyfer AE, Jackson SM. Reduction mammaplasty using the inferior glandular 'pyramid' pedicle: experiences with 300 patients. *Plast Reconstr Surg* 1987; **80**: 75–84.
21. Wise I. Preliminary report of a method of planning the mammoplasty. *Plast Reconstr Surg* 1956; **17**: 367–375.
22. Hoffman S. Recurrent deformities following reduction mammaplasty and correction of breast asymmetry. *Plast Reconstr Surg* 1986; **78**: 55–60.
23. Goldman LD, Goldwyn RB. Some anatomical considerations of subcutaneous mastectomy. *Plast Reconstr Surg* 1973; **51**: 501–505.
24. Woods JE, Irons GB, Arnold PG. The case for submuscular implantation of prostheses in reconstructive breast surgery. *Ann Plast Surg* 1980; **5**: 115–122.
25. Slade CL. Subcutaneous mastectomy: acute complications and long-term follow-up. *Plast Reconstr Surg* 1984; **73**: 84–88.
26. Radovan C. Breast reconstruction after mastectomy using the temporary expander. *Plast Reconstr Surg* 1982; **69**: 195–205.
27. Austed ED, Rose GL. A self-inflating tissue expander. *Plast Reconstr Surg* 1982; **70**: 588–593.
28. Schneider WJ, Hill HL Jr, Brown RG. Latissimus dorsi myocutaneous flap for breast reconstruction. *Br J Plast Surg* 1977; **30**: 277–281.
29. McGraw JB, Dibbell DG, Carraway JH. Clinical definition of independent myocutaneous vascular territories. *Plast Reconstr Surg* 1977; **60**: 341–52.
30. Bostwick J III, Nahai F, Wallace JG, Vasconez LO. Sixty latissimus dorsi flaps. *Plast Reconstr Surg* 1971; **63**: 31–41.
31. Poland A. Deficiency of the pectoralis muscle. *Guy's Hospital Report* 1841; **6**: 191.
32. Hester TR, Bostwick J III. Poland's syndrome: correction with latissimus muscle transposition. *Plast Reconstr Surg* 1982; **69**: 226–33.
33. Hartrampf CR, Scheflen M, Black PW. Breast reconstruction with a transverse abdominal island flap. *Plast Reconstr Surg* 1982; **69**: 216–25.
34. Elliott LF, Hartrampf CR. Tailoring of the new breast using the transverse abdominal island flap. *Plast Reconstr Surg* 1983; **72**: 887–93.
35. Serafin D, Georgiade N. Nipple-areolar reconstruction after mastectomy. *Ann Plast Surg* 1982; **8**: 29–34.
36. Adams WM. Labial transplant for correction of loss of the nipple. *Plast Reconstr Surg* 1949; **4**: 295–298.

# 12

# Psychological manifestations of benign breast disease

J HUGHES

## Introduction

The female breast is an organ of great psychological importance. The appearance of the breasts contributes to a woman's body image and sexual attractiveness. Changes in the breasts occur in relation to menstruation and childbirth, events which may be accompanied by emotional disturbance because of their simultaneous hormonal changes and their psychosocial significance, and cancer of the breast has a widespread reputation as a terrible disease.

Benign breast disease seems likely to have psychological components for all these reasons, but the topic has attracted little scientific research, presumably because cancer of the breast has taken priority. Some of the material in this chapter is therefore based on general principles concerning the psychological aspects of physical illness, rather than on research findings specific to benign breast disease.

The chapter is in three parts: first, a theoretical discussion of the relationship between psychological disorders and benign breast disease, including a selection of case histories to illustrate the various types of link; secondly, a review of published research on the psychological characteristics of patients with benign breast disease; and, thirdly, a practical guide to recognition and management of psychological disorders in patients with benign breast disease.

## Theoretical relationships between psychological disorders and benign breast disease

There is a high prevalence of psychiatric illness, personality disturbance, and social maladjustment among patients who present with somatic symptoms, whether in primary care or general hospitals.[1, 2] Most of the cases of psychological disturbance identified in research surveys appear to be unrecognised and untreated in ordinary clinical practice. There is no simple classification system for these disturbances, and the mechanisms through which they are linked to the somatic symptoms are complex and incompletely understood.

Three main types of link between psychological and somatic disorder can be distinguished, and these will be discussed with special reference to benign breast disease.

## Maladaptive reactions to physical symptoms

The psychological consequences of developing a physical illness range from transient 'adjustment reactions' of an understandable and appropriate kind, to formal psychiatric illnesses requiring specialised treatment. Different physical conditions are distressing in different ways. For patients with benign breast diseases, fear of breast cancer is the cardinal stress. Breast symptoms themselves – for example, mastalgia or nipple discharge – can also provoke psychological disturbance. Extreme reaction patterns of a 'maladaptive' kind[3] include:

*Depression*

This is characterised by lowering of mood, loss of energy, poor concentration, loss of interest, guilt, hopelessness, suicidal thinking, sleep and appetite disturbance.

*Anxiety*

Anxiety is accompanied by constant feelings of dread, inability to relax, insomnia, and symptoms of autonomic disturbance such as palpitations, difficulty in breathing, tremor, sweating, nausea, dysphagia, diarrhoea, and tension headaches.

*Anger*

This sometimes manifests itself as hostile aggressive behaviour towards hospital staff.

*Denial*

There is a lack of concern about potentially serious symptoms, presumed to be an unconscious 'mental mechanism' to protect against anxiety and depression. Denial may lead to delays in consultation or poor treatment compliance.

*Welcoming the 'sick role'*

There is a tendency to exaggerate physical symptoms in order to gain care and attention, or relief from responsibilities. This is usually a genuine expression of distress rather than deliberate malingering.

*Case history: depressive reaction to suspected cancer*

A shop assistant in her late thirties, formerly a contented person who lived happily with her husband and two teenage children, found a lump in her left breast; she felt sure she had breast cancer. Her general practitioner shared her concern and referred her to the breast clinic. She was given an appointment for two weeks later. Throughout this two week period she was acutely depressed, could not eat or sleep, frequently broke down in tears, believed she would die before her children grew up, and was unable to go to work. As soon as she had attended the clinic and been given a diagnosis of benign breast disease, her depressive symptoms cleared up completely.

## Psychological disorders with a somatic presentation

Patients with psychiatric illness, personality disorders, or social difficulties frequently consult their doctors about somatic complaints for which little or no physical basis can be detected. The main conditions likely to present in this way to a breast clinic are:

### Depressive illness

This may give rise to exaggerated fear of serious physical diseases such as cancer, and in extreme cases to hypochondriacal delusions on the same theme.

### Anxiety neurosis

This may also be associated with fears about malignant disease.

### Somatoform disorders

These are physical symptoms for which no organic or physiological basis can be found, but which are accompanied by positive evidence of underlying psychological conflicts.[4] 'Hysterical' and 'hypochondriacal' symptoms are included in this category. Women with minor mood disturbances, vulnerable personalities, social difficulties, or sexual problems may focus their concern on a trivial abnormality of the breast and present this as their main complaint.

### Dysmorphophobia

This is a condition in which the patient believes the appearance of a part of the body is abnormal, although other people consider it unremarkable. Such patients may present to breast clinics with apparently unjustified requests for breast reduction or augmentation.

### Monosymptomatic delusional psychosis

This is a rare condition in which the patient has a fixed false belief of a hypochondriacal kind without other symptoms of psychiatric illness. A conviction of having breast cancer, persisting despite normal investigations and repeated reassurance, would be an example.

### Case histories: hypochondriasis as a symptom of depressive illness

A housewife in her fifties, with a long history of both recurrent major depression and minor surgical operations, had experienced depressed mood, loss of interest in life, lack of energy, pessimism about the future and preoccupation with death (including rumination about suicide) for three months before referral to the breast clinic. Antidepressant drugs had not helped. She told her general practitioner of a small lump in her left breast and asked to be referred to hospital in case this was cancer. At the research interview, however, she admitted the lump had been present unchanged for many years; a lipoma was diagnosed at the breast clinic.

A widow in her sixties had been depressed since her husband's death from bowel cancer eight months earlier. Their only son, who still lived at home, had been off work with 'nerves' since his father died. When this woman found a small lump near her right nipple she was convinced she was going to die from cancer too. Clinical examination at the breast clinic revealed a tiny subcutaneous cyst.

## 'Psychosomatic' disorders

In theory, emotional disturbance could be an aetiological factor for benign breast disease, as the endocrine disturbances known to accompany both depressive illness[5] and stressful life events[6] would be expected to affect breast physiology.

### Case histories: breast lumps developing after psychosocial stress

A secretary in her thirties had been severely depressed for eight months before discovering a breast lump. A hysterectomy for menorrhagia of benign origin had been carried out five months before the lump was found. Difficulties over working conditions had been present for a year; during this time she was dismissed from her job and then reinstated after appealing to an industrial tribunal. At the breast clinic a benign cyst was diagnosed.

A teacher in her thirties moved away from her home town three months before finding a lump in her breast. The move was the result of her husband's wish to change career. The consequences for the patient were largely adverse ones: decreased contact with her parents, giving up her job, taking on renovation of a delapidated house, and a large drop in living standards. She did not become clinically depressed after the move but her physical health deteriorated, with irregular heavy periods and repeated chest infections. The breast lump was diagnosed as fibroadenosis.

A housewife in her fifties was deserted by her husband two years before developing painful lumps in both breasts. She took a job for the first time in 20 years, started divorce proceedings, and put the former matrimonial home on the market. She was menopausal with irregular heavy periods. She had been depressed for several months but the depression had lifted by the time she was referred to the breast clinic, where fibroadenosis was diagnosed.

All three of these patients had menstrual disorders as well as benign breast disease. Menstrual disorders are known to be associated with psychiatric morbidity,[7] although the direction of cause and effect is not clear.

## Research on psychological aspects of benign breast disease

The psychological aspects of benign breast disease have attracted little direct attention. However, patients with such disease have often been used as comparison groups in studies about psychiatric illness, personality characteristics, and life event experience as precursors of breast cancer.[8–18] The usual method has involved interviewing patients who present to hospital with undiagnosed breast lumps; such studies might be expected to yield information about benign breast disease also. Any conclusions about the psychology of either breast cancer or benign breast disease drawn from studies of this kind, however, are likely to be fallacious, because of methodological problems. Any differences found between the two groups of patients might merely refect the likelihood that most patients in both groups have correctly guessed their diagnosis already,[19] even if the interviews were carried out before diagnostic investigations were complete. There is no valid means of comparison with the general population, as the stress of being under hospital investigation for possible malignancy is likely to affect the interview responses of both groups of patients and therefore give a misleading impression of their psychology. Lastly, the breast cancer and benign breast disease groups overlap to some extent, because benign disease is a risk factor for cancer, and because a few early cases of cancer are misdiagnosed as benign breast disease.

The ideal way to overcome these problems would be through large scale prospective studies in the general population, which are time consuming and expensive; it seems feasible, however, to link psychological studies to the new breast screening programmes, and these should succeed in answering most of the criticisms mentioned above.

The results of the various papers[8–18] are summarised in Table 12.1. Variations between the results of different studies exist and may be partly explained by differences in sample selection – for example, were the patients with cancer and benign disease matched for age? was the sample with benign disease drawn from all out-patient attenders or confined to those women admitted for biopsy? Other sources of variation to be considered include: the stage of the diagnostic process at which the interviews were carried out, the questionnaires or diagnostic criteria used for psychometric assessment, the time period that was covered by the interviews, and random variation between small samples.

Pooling the results of these studies does not show any consistent difference between patients with breast cancer and benign disease as regards recent depression, anxiety, or life event experience. A repeated finding, however, is that patients with breast cancer suppress unpleasant emotions such as anger,

**Table 12.1**   Some studies comparing patients with breast cancer and patients with benign breast disease

| First author and year of publication | Number of patients | Summary of findings |
|---|---|---|
| Muslin 1966 | 37   with breast cancer<br>37   with benign disease | No difference in separation experiences during previous three years, or in first nine years of life |
| Greer 1975 | 69   with breast cancer<br>91   with benign disease | Cancer patients showed more suppression of emotion, notably of anger. No difference in extraversion. No difference in depression or life events during previous five years |
| Schonfield 1975 | 27   with breast cancer<br>85   with benign disease | Cancer patients showed greater evidence of 'denial'. Patients with benign conditions had more life events during previous three years. No difference in depression or 'wellbeing'. |
| Maguire 1978 | 75   with breast cancer<br>50   with benign disease | No difference in anxiety or depression before clinic attendance, but more anxiety in cancer patients after attending clinic. |
| Morris 1984 | 17   with breast cancer<br>33   with benign disease | Cancer patients showed greater suppression of anger, less neuroticism, less anxiety. |
| Wirsching 1982 | 18   with breast cancer<br>38   with benign disease | Cancer patients showed more emotional repression, more rationalisation, more optimism, and less anxiety. |
| Jansen 1984 | 69   with breast cancer<br>82   with benign disease<br>71   well women | Patients with benign conditions described as tense, restless, outgoing, and expressing anger. |
| Cheang 1985 | 46   with breast cancer<br>75   with benign disease<br>42   well women | Cancer patients reported more life events during previous two years. Cancer patients more prone to conceal their feelings. |

**Table 12.1** *Cont'd*

| First author and year of publication | Number of patients | Summary of findings |
|---|---|---|
| Priestman 1985 | 100 with breast cancer<br>100 with benign disease<br>100 well women | No difference in life events during previous three years, and no difference in personality measures, between patients with cancer and those with benign conditions. Control group had more life events than either patient group. |
| Hughes 1986 | 33 with breast cancer<br>107 with benign disease | Patients with benign conditions had more major depression and more life events during previous year. |
| Hughson 1987 | 44 with breast cancer<br>47 with benign disease<br>30 after cholecystectomy | Patients with benign conditions had most neuroticism, anxiety, depression, irritability, and loss of libido |

and show low levels of neuroticism, when compared with those with benign disease. Some authors have interpreted this as indicating a true personality difference, and others as evidence of 'denial' by cancer patients who have already guessed their diagnosis. An alternative explanation is that women with benign disease have unusually high levels of neuroticism.

Support for the theory that patients with benign breast disease tend to have high levels of psychological disorder comes from four of the studies.[10, 14, 17, 18] Our Southampton survey[17] was confined to women over 35 referred to the breast clinic with a breast lump as the presenting complaint. Home interviews were carried out a few days before the first breast clinic appointment. The 107 women who subsequently received a diagnosis of benign breast disease were found to have high rates of depression in the year before referral compared with women in published community surveys. This result contrasts with that of a survey of another subgroup of patients with benign disease – those attending a breast clinic for mastalgia[20] – who were not found to have excessive levels of psychiatric disturbance.

Followup studies on breast cancer patients, using patients with benign disease for comparison,[11, 12] show that psychological disturbance in the breast cancer group tends to increase in the months following their referral to hospital, whereas that in the group with benign disease lessens or remains static.

To sum up, there are ample theoretical grounds for supposing that links exist between psychological disorder and benign breast disease but large scale studies to confirm the relationship have not been done.

Whether or not patients with benign disease as a group have a significantly increased incidence of emotional disturbance compared with women in the general population, a number of emotionally disturbed individuals are certainly found in breast clinics and the clinical management of such patients will now be considered.

## Clinical aspects of psychological disturbance in patients with benign breast disease

### Psychological disorder as a determinant of breast clinic referral

Whenever psychological and somatic symptoms coexist, the somatic ones tend to take priority in general practice consultations. This is partly the result of the stigma still attached to emotional disturbance, which often makes both patients and doctors ill at ease when discussing them. A more important factor for somatic complaints involving the breast is the fear of missing a carcinoma. When even the expert cannot make a confident distinction between physiological nodularity and a small malignant lesion by clinical examination alone, false alarms from patients are inevitable and the conscientious general practitioner often feels obliged to arrange a specialist opinion although the breasts seem quite healthy.

Health education about breast self examination and prompt attention to breast abnormalities and the increasing provision of breast screening facilities are obviously commendable if they achieve earlier diagnosis of cancer, but they are also likely to have the undesirable effect of promoting hypochondriacal concern among depressed, anxious, introspective, and unhappy women who have little or nothing wrong with their breasts.

### Psychiatric case detection in the breast clinic

Psychological interviews for all patients with benign breast disease would be neither feasible or desirable, but certain signs should alert the clinician to recognising the more marked cases of psychological disturbance: (a) overt distress in the form of tearfulness, extreme anxiety, or aggression, (b) withdrawn, unresponsive, retarded behaviour, which may mask a severe psychiatric illness such as major depression, and (c) referral, especially repeated referral, in the absence of objective signs of any breast lesion.

A more systematic approach to psychiatric case detection in busy medical and surgical settings is the use of brief self rating questionnaires such as the General Health Questionnaire[22] or the Hospital Anxiety and Depression scale.[23] Patients can be asked to fill in one of these when they arrive at the clinic. Completing and scoring them takes only a few minutes and most patients find the procedure quite acceptable provided its purpose has been tactfully explained. A few sensitive patients, however, will be upset by the implication that their case has psychiatric aspects, and a few will have difficulty completing the form.

In practice, questionnaires tend to be reserved for research purposes. They are a perfectly legitimate means of case detection in clinical settings, but they are not a substitute for personal interview, nor is there any point in using them unless there are facilities for clinical psychiatric assessment of those who obtain high scores.

## Managing psychological disorder in the breast clinic

Because undiagnosed breast symptoms cause so much anxiety, it is desirable that waiting lists be kept short and that patients are informed of investigation results as soon as these are available.

Good staff–patient relationships are always important, and can do much to ameliorate psychological distress of the milder kind. The value of sympathetic listening to patients' concerns, and giving clear explanations about investigations and diagnosis, is easily underestimated. Even if time for talking to patients is limited, it should always be possible to treat them with courtesy and respect. Patients without serious physical pathology, who are likely to be the most psychologically vulnerable, sometimes receive short shrift because they are perceived as wasting clinic time. Belittling their complaints with remarks like 'Your trouble's just in the mind, dear', or 'What you need is a new boyfriend', are patronising at best. At worst, when delivered to a terrified woman by a brusque doctor with an audience of medical students, they can cause lasting distress.

In contrast, when the information that no serious breast disease is present is put over in a firm kindly fashion and accompanied by an explanation of the patient's symptoms she will often be genuinely reassured and go home much happier.

Good staff–patient relationships and simple counselling alone are not sufficient treatment for the more severe psychological disorders, and breast clinic staff seldom have either the time or the skill to treat such cases themselves. Prescribing psychotropic drugs such as benzodiazepine tranquillisers or hypnotics, without a thorough assessment of the psychiatric history and mental state, may do more harm than good.

An ideal course is referral to a specialist. The reasons for this need to be tactfully presented to the patient. Some will be glad that their emotional distress has been recognised and taken seriously, but many people who 'somatise' their emotional complaints readily become indignant if they feel they are being classed as a psychiatric case.

Liaison psychiatrists, nurse counsellors, psychologists, or social workers are sometimes attached to breast clinics, but their prime concern is with the care of breast cancer patients. Providing psychological care for patients with benign disease, who are much more numerous, would require extra facilities on a scale which seems unlikely to be forthcoming in most National Health Service centres at the present time. In the absence of specialist advice in the clinic itself, the best course is to make sure the general practitioner is aware of the psychological difficulties.

## Summary and conclusions

The prevalence of psychological disorder among women with benign breast disease is unknown, but there is ample theoretical reason and some practical evidence to suggest that it is common. For milder cases of benign breast disease, emotional disturbance – often covert – is probably an important determinant of hospital referral; this is an undesirable state of affairs as it diverts clinic facilities from the care of patients with severe benign breast disease or breast cancer without providing full assessment of the primary psychological problems. Existing psychological research studies tend to be confined to special subgroups of benign breast disease, selected as an obvious (though not entirely satisfactory) comparison group for breast cancer patients rather than as subjects of interest in their own right. There is room for larger studies including the whole range of patients with benign breast disease and the introduction of breast screening programmes should facilitate planning of such research.

## References

1. Mayou R, Hawton K. Psychiatric disorder in the general hospital. *Br J Psychiatry* 1986; **149**: 172–90.
2. Lloyd GG. Review article: psychiatric syndromes with a somatic presentation. *J Psychosom Res* 1986; **30**: 113–20.
3. Lloyd GG. Psychological reactions to physical illness. *Br J Hosp Med* 1977; **18**: 352–58.
4. American Psychiatric Association. *Diagnostic and Statistical Manual of Mental Disorders*. 3rd revised ed. Washington DC, American Psychiatric Association, 1987.
5. Ashcroft G. Biochemistry and pathology of the affective psychoses. In: Wing JK, Wing L. (Eds) *Handbook of Psychiatry, Vol 3: Psychoses of Uncertain Aetiology*. Cambridge, Cambridge University Press, 1982.
6. Mason JW. Psychologic stress and endocrine function. In: Sachar EJ. (Ed) *Topics in Psychoendocrinology*. Orlando, Grune and Stratton, 1975.
7. Gath D, Osborn M, Bungay G, *et al*. Psychiatric disorder and gynaecological symptoms in middle aged women: a community survey. *Br Med J* 1987; **294**: 213–18.
8. Muslin HL, Gyarfas K, Pieper WJ. Separation experience and cancer of the breast. *Ann NY Acad Sci* 1966; **125**: 802–06.
9. Greer S, Morris T. Psychological attributes of women who develop breast cancer: a controlled study. *J Psychosom Res* 1975; **19**: 147–53.
10. Schonfield J. Psychological and life experience differences between Israeli women with benign and cancerous breast lesions. *J Psychosom Res* 1975; **19**: 229–34.
11. Maguire GP, Lee EG, Bevington DJ, *et al*. Psychiatric problems in the first year after mastectomy. *Br Med J* 1978; **i**: 963–65.
12. Morris T, Greer S, Pettingale KW, Watson N. Patterns of expression of anger and their psychological correlates in women with breast cancer. *J Psychosom Res* 1981; **25**: 111–17.
13. Wirsching M, Stierlin H, Hoffman F, *et al*. Psychological identification of breast cancer patients before biopsy. *J Psychosom Res* 1982; **26**: 1–10.
14. Jansen MA, Muenz LR. A retrospective study of personality variables associated with fibrocystic disease and breast cancer. *J Psychosom Res* 1984; **28**: 35–42.

15. Cheang A, Cooper CL. Psychosocial factors in breast cancer. *Stress Medicine* 1985; **1**: 61–6.
16. Priestman TJ, Priestman SG, Bradshaw C. Stress and breast cancer. *Br J Cancer* 1985; **51**: 493–98.
17. Hughes JE, Royle GT, Buchanan R, Taylor I. Depression and social stress among patients with benign breast disease. *Br J Surg* 1986; **73**: 997–99.
18. Hughson AV, Cooper AF, McArdle CS, Smith DC. Psychosocial morbidity in patients awaiting breast biopsy. *J Psychosom Res* 1988; **32**: 173–80.
19. Schwarz R, Geyer S. Social and psychological differences between cancer and non-cancer patients: cause or consequence of the disease? *Psychotherapy and Psychosomatics* 1984; **41**: 195–99.
20. Preece PE, Mansel RE, Hughes LE. Mastalgia: psychoneurosis or organic disease? *Br Med J* 1978; **i**: 29–30.
21. Morris T, Greer S, White P. Psychological and social adjustment to mastectomy: a 2-year follow up study. *Cancer* 1977; **40**: 2381–87.
22. Goldberg D. Use of the general health questionnaire in clinical work. *Br Med J* 1986; **293**: 1188–89.
23. Zigmond AS, Snaith RP. The hospital anxiety and depression scale. *Acta Psychiatr Scand* 1983; **67**: 361–70.

# Index